Au Naturel
The History of Nudism in Canada

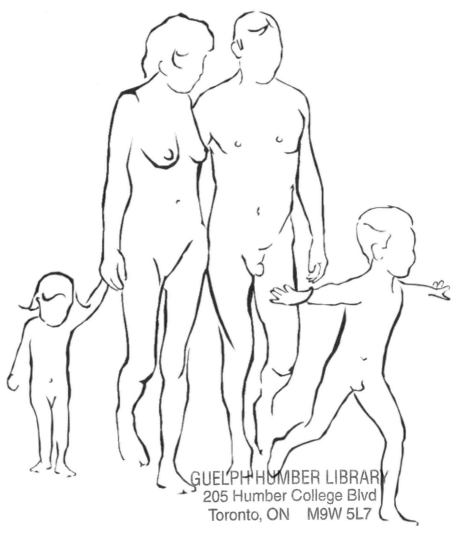

James Woycke, Ph.D.

Published by The Federation of Canadian Naturists
Co-published by Anecdote Productions

National Library of Canada Cataloguing in Publication

Woycke, James Edward, 1947-
    Au naturel : the history of nudism in Canada / James Woycke.

Includes index.

ISBN 0-9682332-3-6

1. Nudism—Canada—History. I. Federation of Canadian Naturists.
    II. Title.

GV451.3.C3W69 2003   613'.194'0971   C2003-901294-8

Editor: John Parry
Cover Design: Ian Cruickshank
Production Supervisor: Stéphane Deschênes

Published by the Federation of Canadian Naturists (FCN)
P.O.Box 186, Stn D, Etobicoke, ON M9A 4X2
www.FCN.ca

Co-published by Anecdote Productions
P.O. Box 81128 FGPO, Ancaster, ON L9G 4X1
www.AnecdoteProductions.com

Printed and bound in Canada by The Aylmer Express Ltd.

PREFACE

Au Naturel is a history of the origin and development of nude recreation in Canada. Tens of thousands of Canadians visit nudist clubs and free beaches in Canada every year, while thousands more visit clubs, resorts, and beaches in the United States, Europe, and the Caribbean, making clothing optional recreation one of the fastest growing sectors of the vacation industry today. How it got that way from its highly individualistic skinny-dipping and sunbathing origins is the story behind *Au Naturel*.

Within the local and regional chapters the sequence of discussion for clubs and beaches is geographical first, then chronological. For example, Chapter Three: Evergreen Tans, starts with a discussion of groups and clubs on Vancouver Island and then proceeds to the Lower Mainland. Chapter Six: Ontario Outdoors, starts with the Toronto area and proceeds to the Golden Horseshoe area, then to Southwest Ontario, then to Central Ontario, and finally to Eastern Ontario. Within each particular region the earliest club is discussed first, followed by later additions.

Au Naturel is based on information from Canadian, American, and European magazines; club and organization newsletters; correspondence between clubs and organizations; reports in the media, and personal interviews. I have quoted liberally from the original sources because the correspondence, records, magazines, and newsletters are not publicly available. I have retained original spelling, grammar, and syntax to reflect the flavor of the original sources. Readers will notice that the endnotes have not been printed here in an effort to hold down the cost of publication. All reference notes will be posted on the FCN web page in summer 2003. [www.fcn.ca/history/endnotes.html.]

Research for this book relied on the free access to sources granted by the Federation of Canadian Naturists, the Fédération québécoise de naturisme, the Western Canadian Sunbathing Association, the Eastern Sunbathing Association, and the American Nudist Research Library. I am grateful to these organizations for their assistance, particularly to Doug Beckett, Michel Vais, Karen Flack, K. Nathesius, and Dot Purcell, respectively, for permission to consult and to quote from these sources. I also want to express general thanks to the various clubs owners, managers, and members who made available club records and correspondence, granted interviews, and otherwise facilitated research. It would be impossible to list everyone here (partly for reasons of confidentiality) but all are acknowledged, however indirectly, in the Notes. And last but certainly not least I owe a tremendous debt to Ray Connett for organizing iv

Canadian nudism in 1947 and seeing it through a very difficult child-hood, and for granting permission to reprint material from his own publications, which are such a vital source for Canadian nudist history. Although Ray (and Mildred) passed away recently, his work lives on in the clubs he founded, both in Canada and in California, and in his tireless work on behalf on nudist organizations in Canada, the United States, and Britain. I also wish to thank the Federation of Canadian Naturists for granting unrestricted access to their papers and to the correspondence and records of the previous Canadian organizations which they have inherited, and for their generous offer to publish this book.

For additional information and resources about nudism/naturism please consult the following resources.

Federation of Canadian Naturists
P.O. Box 186, Station D
Toronto, ON, M9A 4X2
Phone: (416) 410-6833
Fax: (416) 410-6833
Website: www.fcn.ca

Fédération québécoise
de naturisme
4545, avenue Pierre-de-Coubertin
C.P. 1000, Succ. M
Montreal, Quebec, H1V 3R2
Phone: (514) 252-3014
Fax: (514) 254-1363
Website: www.vivrenu.ca

American Association for Nude
Recreation
1703 North Main Street, Suite E
Kissimmee, FL, USA, 34744
Phone: (407) 933-2064
Website: www.aanr.com

The Naturist Society
P.O. Box 132
Oshkosh, WI, USA, 54903
Phone: (920) 426-5009
Website: www.naturistsociety.com

International Naturist Federation
St. Hubertusstraat 5
B-2600 Antwerpen, Belgium
Phone: ++32 3 230 05 72
Fax: ++32 3 281 26 07
Website: www.inffni.org

LIST OF ABBREVIATIONS

AANR	American Association for Nude Recreation (cf. ASA)
AN	Au Naturel (magazine of the FQN)
ANRL	American Nudist Research Library (Florida)
ASA	American Sunbathing Association
BTC	Border Tans Club
CNC	Canadian Nudist Confederation (cf. ECSA)
CND	Camping Nature Détente
CNN	Canadian Nudist News (magazine of the WCSA)
CNRB	Centre Naturiste Richard Brunet
CSA	Canadian Sunbathing Association
CSAir	Canadian Sun Air (continues Sunny Trails magazine)
DNQ	Domaine Naturiste du Québec
ECSA	Eastern Canadian Sunbathing Association
FCL	Forest City Lodge
FCN	Federation of Canadian Naturists
FQN	Federation Québécoise de Naturisme
GHSC	Green Haven Sun Club
GN	Going Natural (magazine of the FCN)
HASS	Health and Sun Society
H&E	Health & Efficiency (British magazine)
INF	International Naturist Federation
LAS	Loisirs-Air-Soleil
LSC	London Sun Club
LST	London Summerset Club
MBC	Meadowbrook Sun Club
MOC	Manitoba Outdoor Club
MTC	Maritan Club
NCC	National Capital Commission
NGS	Niagara Gymnosophical Society
PTC	Paradis Terrestre Club
QTC	Quétans Club
RP	Readers' Page (column in SBH)
SBH	Sunbathing for Health (Canadian magazine)
SBR	Sunny Brae Ranch
SCA	Sunny Chinooks Association
Sgl	Sunglades Club
SH	Sunshine & Health (U.S. magazine)
ST	Sunny Trails (column in SBH)
STC	Sunny Trails Club
SVG	Sun Valley Gardens
STM	Sunny Trails (magazine of the CSA)
SVNP	Sunny Vale Nature Park
TENS	The Edmonton Nudist Society
TGS	Toronto Gymnosophical Society
VTC	Van Tan Club
WCSA	Western Canadian Sunbathing Association
WP	Woman's Page (column in SBH)

TABLE OF CONTENTS

CHAPTER ONE

Bare Beginnings

Some twenty-five years ago, I began my experience in sunbathing. In a small town in Ontario a group of boys would meet on a Saturday morning, fortified by a good healthy picnic lunch, and hike out to the hills, through the bush to the foot of a waterfall. There we would doff our clothes, swim to our hearts content, then lay on the rocks or grass and sunbathe. This is one of my happiest childhood memories.[1]

From coast to coast and at all points in between, from the prairies to the Laurentians, from the Okanagan Valley to Annapolis Valley, virtually all Canadian towns had "the old swimming hole back in the woods a few miles from town" where local boys swam and played nude. "We never dressed from the time we got there until we were ready to go home, so we sure found good health."[2] This skinny-dipping tradition, along with military service and postwar immigration, created favorable conditions for the development of organized social nudism in Canada.

Skinny-dipping meant more than removing a "wet clammy bathing suit" and more than swimming, sunning, and playing nude; it brought a "glorious sense of freedom and vitality and naturalness" that prompted several enthusiasts to wax poetic about answering the "primal call of nature."

> There is something particularly appealing to the young masculine mind about casting off the garb of convention and reverting to the old-fashioned birthday suit. It is more than a mere physical freedom.

> There is something of a subconscious unity with all
> other growing things of nature. One has a feeling of
> belonging to the Divine scheme of existence.[3]

Unfortunately, the "primal call of nature" was intercepted
sometimes by grown-ups with "unscrupulous eyes" who berated
the lads for "swimming with other boys in the nude." But other
youngsters did find parental acceptance—especially if the parents
themselves participated.[4]

When Canadians weren't jumping in the water buck naked
they could often be found lying around the house, the farm, or the
woods soaking up sunshine and fresh air. For these young men
wearing clothes "is just like being tied up." Their preference was
"to get away out in the country and away from everybody and
have a wonderful time all by myself in the good fresh air and sun."
What they did once they got there could be as simple as "to run,
swim, or read a book in the sunshine." The point was to get out
and experience a sunner's high.

> Several years ago I developed the habit of exposing
> my body as much as possible to different conditions,
> to water, sun, and air, and to these natural elements I
> believe that I owe my good health and happy disposi-
> tion."[5]

Men sunbathed whenever they had the opportunity. Road and
railroad workers, lumberjacks, and especially farmers took advantage of isolated locations outdoors to sun while they worked. For
this generation sunbathing combined "healthful relaxation" with
"a nice brown healthy glow" to show for it. Having a tan "as good
as that of an Indian" made them "feel very relaxed and free, like
the happiest person in the world." City dwellers could take
advantage of nude sunning on YMCA roofs (at least in Toronto
and Montreal) or slip off into secluded areas of nearby parks. "I
would go to the back where few people went and there remove my
clothes and sit and relax. More than once I felt like getting up and
running and playing, that was a wonderful summer."[6]

Fresh air was just as important as sunlight for many people. "In the summer when it is nice and warm, I take the boat out on the lake and strip and let the sun and wind caress me and relax me and I drink in the strength that the elements have to offer." Fresh air bathing, unlike sunbathing, could be practiced indoors in complete privacy, after a bath or shower. "My first venture was to open my window, then disrobe completely and enjoy God's gift to humanity." As well, air baths were possible day and night. Many indoor nudists refused to "put clothes on to go to bed" or removed them during the night because "I feel so uncomfortable." Even winter did not deter the true heliophile. One Nova Scotian recalled "being left alone in mid-winter to 'mind the house' for a day and of stripping off my clothes to race about wildly through the knee-deep snow, shouting and laughing with sheer animal joy. Perhaps it is fortunate that our nearest neighbor lived a mile away along the wooded road."[7]

Physical exercise brought a number of young men to nudism, however circuitously. The 1940s and 1950s were the time when Charles Atlas was promising that "in just seven days I can make you a man," while Harold Laurance guaranteed "supermanity" to his followers. Physical culture enthusiasts abounded in Canada. Devotees of Bernarr Macfadden's "physical culture" and of "dynamic tension" embraced nudism as an adjunct to their exercise regimen, even though Ray Connett, the country's foremost nudist writer, downplayed the potential of bodybuilding for promoting nudism because so few Canadians were involved in "athletics and sports." Some bodybuilders incorporated nude exercises into their training regimen at gyms in Montreal and at camps in Canada and Florida, while many more novices did so at home.

> I noticed after training for two or three months that I could derive twice the benefit from my exercises if I were free of hampering clothes and could watch my muscles in motion. The ability to see the portion of the body one is attempting to develop provides, I believe, a great psychological asset to that development.[8]

The purpose of all this elemental exposure and activity was to invigorate the body in order to prevent or cure illness. Sun and air baths were praised as remedies for all sorts of ailments. An arthritis sufferer was advised to get sunlight, which he did while living on a farm, but this ended when "we moved to Copper Cliff and it has been like jail for me." Likewise, men and boys with asthma, heart trouble, nervous disorders, or shingles all credited sunbaths for their improved health. A young spastic who regained movement after walking in the woods got encouragement from his mother, who "made me go in the nude at all times." All of them credited the outdoor life for their success. "Now I am a confirmed sun worshipper and cannot say too much for its healing and healthful powers."[9]

The best thing about the natural road to health was that it was never too late to start. A Winnipegger reported that naturism "has given me health at sixty" after his doctor told him to get more sun because "I was a wreck." But the quintessential—and certainly the most extreme—practitioner of the natural life was Herbert Frank Boyce, who had failed his engineering exams in Britain because of "a nervous breakdown crippling me for nearly two years." He turned to naturopathy and to Canada to restore his health. After chasing Louis Riel he served with the Anglican church before settling in Victoria. When his wife died Boyce moved back to Riel country. He lived in a little log cabin on Ladder Lake near Big River in northern Saskatchewan, wearing only earmuffs in winter while chopping ice for water and hunting for food. In summer he made another cabin available as the Eden Health Resort for like-minded visitors. "In my naturistic home I am quite well and happy, free from colds and other ailments to which a man of my age (73) might be subject." Boyce died in 1952.[10]

Outdoor recreation—hiking, camping, canoeing—provided ideal opportunities for groups of boys or men to enjoy nude swimming or sunning at isolated lakes, beaches, rivers, and woods across Canada. "Almost every year a group of boys and I have been going up north to Algonquin Park for two weeks where we enjoy many happy hours swimming nude." Summer camp, including church and scout camps, offered a more organized introduction to "skin swims" for many boys.

> As a Cubmaster I have held camps of my own this past year and encouraged the young lads to romp in the sun with little or no clothing. . . . When we take our hikes in summer there is always a stream or river nearby for swimming and the youngsters really enjoy it.[11]

What's sauce for the gander is sauce for the goose: girls and women also enjoyed skinny dipping and sunbathing, in either mixed or all-female groups; rarely alone, although one man reported that in his line of work he noticed "an amazing number of women who are practicing nude sunbathing on house roofs, screened porches, etc." Girls attending summer resorts in vacation districts like the Muskokas sometimes hiked out to relatively secluded spots where they "discard all clothing and swim and play. . . . I came upon such a scene last year quite unexpectedly, but the group had been warned . . . and there they all lay, on their tummies, towels thrown across their backs. They just lay there and all stared at me, and I smiled and kept on my way." Another young man, sunbathing nude at Mary Lake, was pleasantly surprised when two girls walked by on the beach—also nude. Elsewhere in northern Ontario a group of girls had exclusive use of a cottage for much of the summer of 1939, where "we spent long hours in the sun after bathing in the clear water."[12]

Once introduced to nudism, girls became quite assertive. Two young guests at a northern resort asked one of the young men to row them out to an island. "As soon as they climbed ashore they stripped off their clothes and asked me to join them. I never forgot the pleasure of being so free out in the open." In some of the small towns around the country the local water hole was used by all ages and genders, albeit under a strict protocol whereby males and females undressed and entered the water at different spots, and then "we all swam and romped together."[13]

When these young men and women married they faced the

challenge of converting a reluctant or inexperienced spouse, or else dropped out of nudism. Some women "soon discovered the wonderful freedom and healthfulness of nudism." Whether from attraction—"I became interested through the boyfriend and believe me he certainly shows the benefit of sunbathing"—or shared interest—"we sleep nude, swim nude, and go without clothes whenever we can"—wives and girlfriends often joined their partners in the sun.[14]

Families who share a commitment to nudism make it a part of their everyday lives as much as possible by way of "domestic" nudism. This might mean sleeping without pyjamas, or relaxing nude at the end of the day—"Oh, what pleasure, after work, in the evening to get out of one's clothes and to feel free"—or going without clothes completely while at home: "Clothes are the last thing we think of." But nudism is best enjoyed outdoors, so couples sought "a secluded spot in the countryside," or took a "naturist holiday" camping on isolated lakes "where we could go nude at any time." Still others preferred to canoe and sail through the "wave-washed islands" of Georgian Bay "in tune with our surroundings."[15]

The family cottage was the most convenient location for nude vacations for the whole family, and sometimes for their friends.

> As soon as we got there the children were allowed to romp about in or out of the water completely naked . . . . Those were happy times for me, and I do not remember ever being healthier than during the three summers my friends included me in their outings.[16]

But as the increasing pressure on cottage country made it "hard to find a place where we can catch a bit of sun . . . not with those curious people crawling around," resourceful couples coped by "swimming . . . in the moonlight" or by waiting until off-season, "when the beaches were deserted and we were able to experience the freedom of being nude." Others found safety in numbers. "My wife and I have experienced naturism a few times in the past when we used to go bathing for the day with a mixed group at a summer cottage." Here and there across Canada small groups gathered at isolated cottages or private camps for swimming, fishing, or tennis. "We all feel so at home in our group at the cottage."[17]

All this romping and frolicking in the great outdoors carried with it the risk of discovery by "berry pickers, hikers, and so forth." A gentleman emerging from Lake Erie found himself accosted by an irate young man and woman who threatened court action and demanded his name, which he cheerfully provided: "I wonder just what he will do when he appears in court and finds that I am the judge of this district?" But not all the intruders were hostile. One young man cavorting in the Bay of Quinte on Lake Ontario attracted the attention of a boatload of fisherfolk. When he came out of the water and lay on the beach one of the men followed him and asked if they could join him, "as I looked so carefree and healthy." In British Columbia a couple working in the Caribou area fell asleep after a skinny dip in the river, only to be awakened by voices. The husband got his swim suit on but his wife couldn't decide between the top or the bottom of hers and ducked behind him. Then they both laughed when they saw that their visitors were a family of eight and that "all the clothing between them was a pair of shorts on the second oldest girl and a pair of sandals on the feet of the mother." And two brothers camping at Loon Lake in Ontario converted three other teens when a family came across the brothers sunning nude. Although the mother "sure laid into us," the parents left their children behind with the boys. "They were real nudists as it turned out, so we had two weeks that I call "swell.""[18]

However enjoyable, skinny-dipping and sunbathing were lonely pleasures for the early generations of Canadian nudists. Individuals, small groups, and families cavorted in isolation, unaware that their pastime had a name and a history and—elsewhere—an organization. The Second World War and postwar immigration wave introduced social nudism to Canadians.

Military service in the Second World War exposed thousands

of Canadians to societies where nudism was more widespread, better organized, and more socially accepted than in their own benighted Dominion. "I really believe that the last war has changed the views of many towards greater freedom in sun-bathing and swimming free of all clothing." For some, revelation came simply from meeting other Canadians from all parts of the country and finding that "there were thousands of people thinking like me." These like-minded individuals set about swimming and sunning while in training.[19] Service personnel who trained in Ontario were made welcome by members of the Sun-Air club, which rented island camps in Georgian Bay and the Kawarthas.

> Pulling on the oars in the last lap of the journey to the island rendezvous . . . we were astounded to find a strange flotilla indeed coming out to meet us—a veritable fleet bearing down on us in review order with large Union Jacks unfurled in the breeze. The fact of the fleet being composed of a sailboat, a rowboat, and a canoe, all filled to capacity with enthusiastic Sun-Air-Freedom Lovers lustily chanting a song of welcome, did not detract from the grandeur of the occasion. As both my companion and myself were wearing the uniform of the Armed Services the significance of this welcome will be long remembered.[20]

For other servicemen it was assignment in Europe that provided their first contact with nudism. "I was Overseas for five years in World War II and had the pleasure over there of nude bathing and sunbathing, and believe me, no one knows the thrill of this type of life who has not tried it." Canadians usually found themselves posted to England before shipping out to combat theaters in North Africa, Sicily, France, Holland, and Germany.[21]

In England Canadians had "the wonderful opportunity to visit and become a member of many a club." Spielplatz, Heritage, North Devon, and the Arcadians—proud home of a German bomb crater—were just a few of the British clubs that opened their doors to "lone Canadian nudists" and provided a "wonderful place to go for a real rest." One Canadian even found himself boarding with fellow nudists, while others bunking together in barracks practiced indoor nudism as a means to "overcome colds and the English climate." In North Africa and Italy soldiers would search for a cool spot for swimming as a break from the tropical heat.[22]

In liberated Europe, Canadians encountered continental clubs even older than their British counterparts. They also found greater tolerance of nudity than prevailed in either England or Canada. Occasionally their own Military Police sometimes dragged them back to base and filed charges of "indecent appearance in public," which sympathetic superior officers promptly dismissed.[23]

After the war British and continental nudism influenced Canadians in another way: through immigration. Many new arrivals had some sort of naturist experience, whether in the Scouts—"I have often played and enjoyed swimming in the nude at Gilwell Park, the Boy Scout camping center in England"—the British YMCA, or simply skinny-dipping in the countryside. Other newcomers had experience with mixed skinny-dipping or with nude swimming in the tropics before and during the war. Many were members of the same British nudist clubs that had welcomed Canadian servicemen. But few could match the experience of R.K. of Winnipeg. As a boy he grew up in a family which practiced domestic nudism "purely because we liked the free, relaxed feeling," and "scrubbed my mother's back in the bath and thought nothing of it." As a teenager he worked as a stagehand in the Windmill Theatre, "a sort of refined burlesque show," featuring tableaux vivants "with all those nude or nearly nude models." As a young man he joined Spielplatz as a jack of all trades and led "an idyllic life—working, sleeping, and playing in the sun." And as a pilot in the Royal Air Force during the Berlin air lift of 1948 he commuted between British and German sun clubs. Now the New World beckoned. "My sincere hope is to go, in Canada, helping if I can, the movement which has helped me to health and happiness."[24]

New Canadians from the continent also had experience with naturism. For Europeans, too, skinny-dipping and sunbathing were part of growing up, whether in France, Holland, or Scandinavia, on the Baltic, the Mediterranean, or a snowcapped mountain in Greenland, where workers "took off our clothes and sunbathed lying on the snow." Germany—homeland of many new Canadians who became club leaders and members—had the unique heritage of the Wandervogel youth groups which practiced communal nudism.

> In Germany I belonged to a youth movement where swimming in the nude was quite common. Over the weekends girls and boys cycled together to rivers and lakes where we knew for sure the possibility of strange people seeing us practicing nudism was very unlikely. There it was that I received my first experience of swimming and sunbathing in the nude. It sure was a nice time we boys and girls had together, and I still enjoy those hours in my thoughts.[25]

Not all youthful experiences were this carefree, of course; beaches in the Balkan and Mediterranean countries were segregated by gender. But in every case skinny dipping left a lasting impression that prompted newcomers to seek contact with like-minded Canadians. "I would like to share the fun with others who are of the same mind. To talk and have games with men and women, boys and girls, all in our natural uniform, has been my desire for some time."[26]

Some Europeans learned of nudism while serving in their own armed forces during the war. A German soldier's sunbathing diary reads like a Baedecker guide to combat theaters: "on the coast of Greece, on the Black Sea in Romania, on the Danube in Bulgaria, on the Adriatic Sea in Yugoslavia and Italy, on the Dnieper River in Russia, and after the war in Germany on the North Sea." For some Europeans on the Allied side the fighting did not all stop in 1945, nor did the nudism. Combatting national independence movements in the tropical colonies introduced still more young men to nudism.[27]

Many new Canadians had been members of nudist clubs in

France, Germany, and Austria. The Lobau park in Vienna evoked fond memories: "I spent four years with this big family of nudists and I can say it was the happiest and healthiest time of my life." Others had visited nude beaches in Germany, Scandinavia, Yugoslavia, and the famous Ile du Levant on the French Riviera. For all Europeans aware of the cultural differences between the old country and the new there was a sense of urgency in their desire to join a Canadian club "before I become engulfed in the prevailing Victorian attitudes of this province."[28]

Canadians benefitted from the development of American nudism during the 1930s, 1940s, and 1950s and visited many of the established clubs south of the border. In the West the main destinations included Cobblestone Suntanners, Fraternity Snoqualmie, and the Hesperions in the Pacific Northwest; and Elysia, Olympic Fields, Oakdale Ranch, and Samagatuma in California. In the East Canadians visited Fernglades and the Solair Recreation League in New England; Camp Goodland and Sunshine Park in New Jersey; Gro-Tan, Halcyon, Penn-Sylvan, Pine Tree, Sunny Rest in the Mid-Atlantic states; Lake of the Woods and Zoro Nature Park in Indiana; Sunshine Gardens in Michigan; and—an early favorite for snowbirds—Lake Como in Florida.

> Then I discovered this "real garden of Eden." We stayed a week—the rest of our holidays. The kids were happy, the food was frugal, but excellent. They were free to run around and there were kids to play with. Their parents relaxed and had the wonderful opportunity to be introduced to a new philosophy of living. We played, we bathed, we walked through beautiful gardens.[29]

Canadians and new Canadians alike depended on American, British, and European nudist magazines for information on naturism. "The real impetus for nudism in Canada was the sale of the English totally retouched nudist magazine, Health and Efficiency, on many Canadian newsstands." H&E led Canadians to the American Sunbathing Association and Sunshine and Health, which led them to Ray Connett and his "Canada Speaks" column, and thence to the Canadian magazine Sunbathing for Health, which became the cornerstone of the Canadian Sunbathing Association. "What there is of the Canadian nudist movement probably owes its existence to this magazine."[30]

Sunbathing and Health, later *Sunbathing for Health*, was published in Toronto from May 1939 to March 1959 by the Health Publications Company, later Anglo-American News and then the Rex Book Company, all owned and operated by Thomas Harold Sinnott, president of Sinnott News Company, a large-scale newspaper and magazine distributor. Every month the magazine presented an array of articles on health and hygiene (from a naturopathic perspective), physical culture, figure photography, nature articles on "little birds and bees," and (occasionally) reports on nudism and nudist clubs in England and Europe.[31]

Access to nudist magazines was not always possible in the early years. Ray Connett lamented that "a guardian government protects us from the defilement of nudist news in American and British magazines." Virtually all the principal foreign magazines—*American Nudist Leader, Health and Efficiency, Sun Bathing Review, Sunshine and Health, Vivre d'Abord*—were banned in Canada at one time or other, either by federal Customs and Postal authorities or by local police action as in Ottawa in 1948. But the bans were neither uniform nor permanent, and there was always the option of cross-border shopping.[32]

Unfortunately, even the Canadian magazine, *Sunbathing for Health*, was banned on about half of the newsstands in English Canada, and all of the newsstands in Quebec. It was even banned in its home town: "since moving to this hick town my reading was cut off, since they don't allow it sold on the newsstands of Toronto." And the Post Office withheld mailing privileges. The reason for the ban was moralistic opposition to the nude pictures.

> I've never seen such a horrible paper in my life. This should be taken to the law and to run you out of town.

You must really enjoy yourself taking such pictures.
Why in the world if you have such places can't you
keep them quiet, or do you like looking at the naked
women so much? All I can say is you are pretty rot-
ten.[33]

Nudists themselves expressed concern over the pictures, not
because of the nudity but because of the unrepresentative character of that nudity. "We feel that you do not give a true picture
of nudists by publishing all the very fine-figured girls and Atlas
type men." One random count by a reader showed twenty-eight
pictures of "nude girls and women" but only five of "men with
loin covers." Other readers complained that the magazine
depicted few children and older nudists, thereby neglecting the
family orientation of social nudism. "It would be fatal for men
and women who are somewhat older and considering extending
nudity beyond the home to be forced to the belief that it was
entirely a matter of physique or just something for young
people."[34]

The "false" pictures and the "foul" advertisements caused
many nudists and non-nudists to question the motivation of readers who bought nudist magazines. The suspect readers included
girls who presumably followed the exploits of the Atlas-type
physique models, and "young single men who no doubt are looking for a thrill at seeing a nude figure."[35]

The photographs used in *Sunbathing for Health* reflected supply
more than demand. Most of the "Venus-type" young women were
artist models, many of them photographed by Blake McLachlan, a
Toronto real estate agent who sold the prints to Sinnott. He also
wrote a series of articles on photography for the magazine. Most
of the pictures of the "Atlas type" physique models were also sup-
plied commercially by the Lanza studio in Montreal and by Earl
Forbes in New York. When real nudist scenes were featured they
were likely to be borrowed from English or European magazines,
since Canadian clubs remained reluctant to supply pictures to a
public magazine.[36]

Nudists also objected to the graphic retouching of photographs to conceal the pubic area. Both males and females were "mutilated" but in different ways. The men had a "ridiculous black pouch" painted over their pubic area, even if the genitals were not visible in the original picture, while the women had the entire pubic area airbrushed out of existence—all because "we must bow down to the guardians of our morals." This retouching did not unduly disturb dedicated nudists, who saw in the pictures "superior beings, whose ideals and morally clean minds, are miles above those who live the so-called 'normal life'." But the alterations might create a misleading impression among novices who read about nude-ism but saw only males in posing straps and females with cleanly shaven pubic areas (which was a trend in some British and American clubs at the time).[37]

Connett argued that Sinnott's magazine, *Sunbathing for Health*, with its suggestive pictures and sensationalist advertising, was a necessary evil. "Yes, his magazine is sexy, yes, it is bought primarily for curiosity by lower class prospects." But it was the only game in town, the only commercially distributed Canadian nudist magazine available to the general public. "Out of it has come all that we call nudism in Canada today, and don't ever forget that." So even though he deplored "the misuse of our illustrations by curiosity seekers," even though the magazine "is forbidden in nearly half the news stands of our land" and sold sub rosa "among the girlie-girlie sex trash" at "skid road dives, pool halls, and cheap cigar stands," Connett remained convinced that pictures were vital for selling nudism: "we must have a means of contacting the general public."[38]

Connett further argued that the "right sort of prospect" who might have bought the magazine for "different reasons than I am writing now" would "go on to read and become interested in our way of life," as some did.

> I have just read your publication for the first time. I didn't even buy it, but read a copy that my roommate had acquired somewhere. I think I am a normal

young man with a healthy mind. When I picked up
your magazine it was only to look at the pictures. It
was sometime later that I took the trouble to read the
printed material.[39]

The problem that did concern Connett was the "fools" who
traded nude pictures through the mails—something that was illegal in Canada and the United States and which jeopardized the
standing of bona fide clubs, organizations, and magazines. He
became especially upset when the "fools" wrote to him asking for
original prints of some of the pictures in *Sunbathing for Health* on
spurious grounds: amateur photographers who wanted unretouched pictures "as study subjects"; neighbors who "used to live
near" one of the models and who requested "the unretouched pho-
tograph of her" for old times' sake; and novices who wanted to
convince a hesitant wife or daughter and thought that "photos of
young girls—in which one can see all parts of their bodies—would
make them see and appreciate the merits of your splendid way of
life."[40]

The Canadian Sunbathing Association had an ambivalent relationship with its mentor magazine from the birth of the CSA to the
death of the magazine (which incidentally coincided with the
death of the CSA as a national organization). At the founding convention in 1947 delegates criticized *Sunbathing for Health* on
account of the "foul" advertising in the magazine, and this
remained a concern for years. It seemed to many as though nudism was just a sideline to fill space between the pages of ads for
"sensational books" such as *Sinful Cities of the Western World*,
Casanova's Memoirs, *The Torch of Life* (the "best methods of consum-
mating the sexual union"), and various "true confessions" of pros-
titutes, dope fiends, and other "vice addicts." But Sinnott ignored
the repeated complaints of CSA officials because the "sensational
books" were his bread and butter, and Connett discouraged other
officials from protesting too much because the magazine provided
his bread and butter too. Everyone who replied to his "Sunny
Trails" column or to the "Woman's Page" received promotional
material for magazine subscriptions. And, as he never tired of

pointing out, the magazine was the bread and butter of the CSA and of all nudist clubs as well: "95% of all our present contacts came to us through that medium, questionable or undesirable as it may be."[41]

As late as November 1958 the Western Division of the CSA reiterated its opposition to the "girlie-girlie" photos which "did not depict the true picture of Canadian nudism." Then the publisher announced that he would stop producing *Sunbathing for Health* at the end of the year (the March 1959 issue), and suddenly the CSA changed its tune. They now admitted that the magazine they had reviled for years was, as Connett had always argued, "the main source of all applications for membership." They now conceded, when it was too late, that "it does a very fine job for nudism in Canada," and they admitted that "if we tire of its posed models we must remember that the magazine is a commercial enterprise and that it must fill its pages to keep up its circulation."[42]

In Toronto officials of the CSA Eastern Division met with Mrs. Sinnott, who seemed more sympathetic to their concerns and who promised "all the cooperation possible." But the bottom line was that the magazine was losing nearly $1,000 per issue, thanks to competition from real "girlie-girlie" magazines like Playboy which satisfied the market for "bare bosoms" better in "glorious technicolor" than *Sunbathing* could with tired old black and white.[43]

With the demise of *Sunbathing for Health* in 1959 the Canadian need for an American magazine on the newsstands became urgent. At the same time the government initiated a review of the obscenity provisions in the Criminal Code. This initiative happened to coincide with a recent U.S. Supreme Court decision clearing nudist magazines of obscenity charges. As a result, *American Sunbather*, *Modern Sunbathing*, and a host of other nudist magazines soon became available in Canada. And in 1962 Canada Customs authorized CSA members to receive unretouched nudist magazines such as Nude Living and Sundial, published in California by Ed Lange. But by this time Playboy and its imitators had made a mockery of bureaucratic concerns with nudist magazines. Unfortunately, they also made the nudist magazines of the 1960s a mockery of true nudism.

> The nudist magazines still bring enquiries. However, they no more are sociological and scientific publications as they used to be. They have degenerated right down into the gutter with all the other pornography selling nudity and sex, not nudism as we practice it. The sooner the authorities step in and clean them up the better.[44]

The Canadian skinny-dipping and sunbathing experience, wartime exposure to American and European nudism, postwar immigration, and access to nudist magazines led thousands of Canadians to embrace social nudism. Together they founded, joined, and developed dozens of nudist clubs across Canada.

CHAPTER TWO

Getting Started

R ay Connett is the man who, in his own humble words, "start-ed the whole nudist movement in Canada." Connett (the name "rhymes with cadet not bonnet") was born and raised in Saskatchewan, where his only introduction to nudism was a chance remark by his father one day in the barn: "wouldn't it be nice if people were so decent inside themselves that it didn't mat-ter to them whether they wore clothes or not?" Connett married Mildred Harris in Calgary, and they moved to Vancouver in 1934. On a cross-border shopping trip to Bellingham, Washington, he noticed a copy of the American magazine *The Nudist* (later renamed *Sunshine and Health*), which he bought and "smuggled" into Canada. He also read the British magazine *Health and Efficiency*, which made him aware of the National Sun-Air Association in England, so when he saw a small personals ad in the local paper announcing the formation of a similar group in Vancouver he replied eagerly. Hardy and Lenore Kaye and a handful of others formed the Van Tan Club, now the oldest club in Canada.[1]

In August 1939 there was more than Pacific rain clouds on the horizon, and Connett like many other Canadians enlisted in the army. After training in signals on Vancouver's Tower Beach (his first exposure to Wreck Beach), Connett was off to Ontario for training at Camp Borden and the Royal Military College before shipping out to England in 1941. He eventually saw service in Italy, and returned home in 1945.

Connett's time in England shaped his future nudist career. "Long ago in wartime England, when friendly clubs made a lone

Canadian nudist welcome, the dream was born, the idea that someone must take up the cause of nudism in Canada." Connett carried with him letters of introduction from the Kayes to the Arcadians of Sun Hill, a club near London which later became the North Kent Sun Club. Through them he met the editor of the *Sun Bathing Review* and started writing articles on Canada and the United States, while also submitting articles and pictures on England to *Sunshine and Health* and to *Sunbathing for Health*, whose publisher he had met in Toronto in 1941.[2] Connett also visited the Heritage and North Durham clubs, and in 1943 he participated in the founding meeting of the British Sun Bathing Association "in the back of a little tea shop in the shadow of the British Museum." Even on active duty Connett found time for nudism in the fields and hills and beaches of Italy, and urged his fellow soldiers to keep their "freedom from inhibition" alive after the war. "My experience abroad strengthened a determination to see nudism grow in strength and power in Canada."[3]

Back home in Vancouver, Connett rejoined the Van Tans and caught up on wartime developments in the ASA. In 1946 he attended the founding meeting of the Northwest Conference, a regional grouping of ASA clubs in the Pacific Northwest, at the Cobblestone Club in Yelm, Washington. This event, along with his British experience, inspired him "to do the same for all of Canada."[4]

By now Connett was convinced that publicity was the key to everything. On his return from England he had stopped at the office of *Sunbathing for Health* in Toronto to renew contact with the publisher, whom he had met while training in Ontario. Connett offered to write a regular column of Canadian content with news, feature articles, and a directory of clubs—all patterned after the *Sunshine and Health* model. The publisher, T.H. Sinnott, accepted the proposal in summer of 1946, and the "Sunny Trails" column was born (the name "came to mind," and Connett stuck with it, using it for his own newsletter/magazine and his own nudist club).[5]

In the December 1946 issue of *Sunbathing for Health* Connett asked plaintively, "is there a nudist in the house?" Recounting his meetings in England and in the United States, where he was constantly asked "what about nudism in Canada," and recalling his wartime conversations with fellow Canadians where he learned of furtive groups in Edmonton, Regina, and Toronto in addition to his own Vancouver club and neighboring Victoria group, Connett wondered: "maybe there are nudists in Canada, maybe there aren't, and he asked his readers to let him know."[6]

By May 1947 Connett had reports on half a dozen clubs and groups from across Canada. His own club, the Van Tans, led the way. Jim Sewell of Victoria confirmed the existence of a group on Vancouver Island, "so we are not doing so badly on the Pacific Coast at any rate." At the northern end of the island, Jack started the Silver Sands Club of Sointula, on Malcolm Island. Other sun-bathers from the "wonderful Okanagan Valley" replied, touting the sun, the lakes, and the scenery of the B.C. Interior.[7]

A couple from Edmonton and a widower from Calgary opened up the prospect of activity in Alberta. A small group in Whitehorse checked in. A family in Sarnia became the Friendship Club, while other Ontarians reported from Guelph, Hamilton, Kingston, Kitchener, and London. One of the most promising responses came from North Bay, where Bob Babcock had been "an ardent sun fan" for some time, and would soon join the Sun Air club in Ontario.[8]

Several people from Atlantic Canada replied to Connett's plea, including the conductor of an "All-Girl Orchestra" in Halifax, who gathered several interested singles and couples for indoor winter gatherings, where "we had a great time," and for summer outings on an island in St. Margaret's Bay that were "gratifying and successful." But the press of business kept the Haligonians from organizing a club, so the job of starting the first nudist club in Atlantic Canada fell to Marcus Meed of New Brunswick, whom Connett described as "one of the strongest, most ardent nudists in all of Canada" and who "deserves a page all by himself."[9] This is it.

Meed was born and raised in Bristol, New Brunswick—a small town on the St. John River in the heart of McCain country. Apart from a few wanderyears in the 1920s—during which time he embraced the philosophy of nudism—Meed spent his life in Bristol. He took over his father's business—Meed's Machine Shop—and he was active on the town council and the school board, in the local church, and in community life generally. He founded both a square dancing club and a summer Bible camp, and in 1984 he wrote a centennial history of Bristol, *Of Interest to Recall.*[10]

During the war years (when he was denied enlistment because of age), Meed secured war contract business in his machine shop and travelled frequently to Ottawa. It was on one of these trips that he obtained copies of *Sunbathing for Health*, came into contact with the Sun Air Freedom Lovers, and thus became one of the respondents to Connett's article when he replied: "emphatically, yes, there is a nudist in Canada." Meed later supported the formation of the Canadian Sunbathing Association in 1947, where his dedication and common sense led to his election as CSA president in 1949. When this was reported in his home town—"a small village, possibly 600 inhabitants, with maybe 100 very vocal Mother Grundys"—one respected church member called him over to report that "when I heard what some of your neighbors are saying I told them that Marcus was not doing something shady or immoral."[11]

For several years Meed tried to organize nudists in Atlantic Canada, but he was hampered by the illness of his wife, who received all his attention, and by his own operation for a brain tumor in 1950. None the less the Atlantic Recreational Club gathered names and in 1955 several devotees met at Meed's private camp just outside Bristol to set up regular operation. "Every one is a real lady or gentleman, a good mixer, and a lasting friend." A year later they drafted a constitution and renamed themselves the Maritans. The club affiliated with the CSA and the ASA.[12]

Meed's club used an abandoned lumber camp. It had 140 acres

of bush land with a spring-fed pond that provided swimming for all "till Joe lost his balance. The pool has seemed quite shallow since that great splash." Other facilities included a clubhouse and cabins; volleyball and badminton courts; archery, ping pong, and croquet; and a children's playground with swings, merry go round, and wading pool. At its peak forty adults and almost as many children belonged to the Maritans.[13]

In 1960 Meed's wife, Evelyn, died. By this time his sons were grown and living away (two later moved back), and many club members who were in the Armed Forces found themselves reassigned elsewhere. In 1963 the Maritans ceased operation on an organized basis, although friends remained welcome at the camp, and Meed stayed in touch with the Eastern Canadian Sunbathing Association for several years. But there would be no other Maritimes club until after Meed's death in 1985, despite attempts in 1968 to form the Seaboard International Gymnosophical Society.[14]

As this preliminary survey indicates, what started as a small trickle of isolated responses soon became a wave of 500 replies which Sinnott forwarded to Connett at his own expense. In return Ray advised these people to subscribe to *Sunshine and Health*, "much better a magazine." He also compiled a "Directory of Groups Forming," although "only four groups in all of Canada" were solidly established.[15]

To accommodate these "oh-so-shy" nudists, Connett started producing the "Sunny Trails" newsletter in the spring of 1947 as a medium of information and an aid to organization. On its pages he listed biographical profiles from individuals who wrote to him and who were willing to contact others in their home area. The response was enormous: there were "hundreds of keen alert young men who were taking sun baths and swimming in the nude but who had never guessed there were actually clubs in Canada or people like themselves anxious to start clubs."[16]

Later that year (1947) Connett started another publication, the

Canadian Nudist Registry, as a "top secret" directory that contained nothing but personal blurbs from individuals willing to contact others—a "correspondence club for nudists." The Registry was sold only to nudists or to sympathizers who were listed in it themselves. "Its chief value and benefit is to those who live at a considerable distance from any club. It provides the means for nudists and prospective nudists to meet each other and arrange outings." But the directory became more than a forum for nudist pen pals. "Many people join the Registry for the sole purpose of collecting nude pictures. They are not nudists, but more or less perverts." Connett reluctantly conceded that "the people in it are not necessarily bona fide nudists," and the Registry itself contained a notice asking members to forward "objectionable" letters from contacts. He himself reported several picture traders to postal authorities in Canada and the United States, but disavowed any responsibility for the "perverts."[17]

In the end, however, it was his regular column in *Sunbathing for Health* that served to unite nudists in Canada and to advise them on starting and developing nudist clubs. For this work Connett drew on his experience with American and British clubs, organizations, and publications, but he often found himself stymied by the resistance of the "oh-so-shy" Canadians to bold initiatives that had proven successful elsewhere. "I have my own ideas, but for the most part if they appeared in print they would merely serve to antagonize existing groups." His uphill battle in his home club, the Van Tans, was proof of this.[18]

When social nudism started to develop clubs across Canada in the 1940s the process was much more complicated than it would be later. For one thing the CSA constantly had to assure people that nudism was indeed legal. The Criminal Code of Canada first defined nudity as an offense in 1931 in response to the protest tactics of the Sons of Freedom sect of the Doukhobors, which involved ritual stripping to demonstrate shame during legal proceedings. In 1953-54 the Criminal Code was amended and all references to "parading" were removed. Section 205A became Section 154, later Section 170 (in 1970) and now Section 174.

> Every one who, without lawful excuse,
> (a) is nude in a public place, or
> (b) is nude and exposed to public view while on private property, whether or not the property is his own, is guilty of an offense punishable on a summary conviction.

Throughout the course of these revisions, two elements of the original law have been retained: the notional definition that "a person is nude who is so clad as to offend against public decency or order," and the limiting condition that "no proceedings shall be commenced under this section without the consent of the Attorney General." The law prohibits nudity in a public place, or nudity on private property while a person is exposed to public view. Conversely, the law permits nudity on screened private property or on secluded public property.

> *There is no law against nudism in Canada . . . providing* you practice it in private. . . . You may sunbathe, swim, play games, one person or one hundred persons, all nude, provided you do it in strict privacy.[19]

The Canadian Sunbathing Association, formed in 1947, recommended a standard procedure for recruiting and organizing members of new clubs, which Connett explained at length in a series of articles in *Sunbathing for Health*. The procedure involved recruiting local organizers, attracting potential members, and bringing both parties together to start a club.

Nudist magazines with national circulation were crucial in this first step. Both *Sunbathing for Health* and *Sunshine and Health* carried lists of clubs, groups forming, and district organizers, depending on the number of known enthusiasts in each location. Readers who were persuaded by the articles and pictures to try social nudism wrote to the magazine, and Connett forwarded their letter to the appropriate address, hoping—sometimes against hope—that the club organizers would reply.[20]

Over time organizers came to rely on advertising in the personal or classified sections of local newspapers, while established clubs invited reporters to visit and write about them, which provided free publicity and implicit approval. But many editors refused to accept ads for nudism in their hallowed family papers, so the CSA advised clubs to use euphemisms such as sunbathing, sun club, or sun-air outings, as well as code words such as "members of ASA or BSBA wish to form club," which would attract the initiate but not the novice. However, Connett argued against using the "weasal word" naturism because its elastic meaning, covering everything from bird watching to vegetarianism, would only confuse people, as indeed it sometimes did.

> I have a feeling that organized nudists are, shall we
> say, composed of a fair percentage of cranks, diet fad-
> dists, 100% anti-alcoholists, strict non-smokers,
> spending half the day doing exercises.[21]

Step Two involved coaching the organizers and the applicants. The ideal group leaders would be a married couple or family with a strong commitment to the philosophy and practice of social nudism. Once prospects wrote in, organizers responded with information sheets, brochures, and an invitation to arrange a meeting hosted by the organizers. There, in the comfort and civility of their home, with an array of nudist material at hand to document and illustrate social nudism for novices, each party could assess the other to decide whether they were right for each other. Leaders had to be on their best behavior lest they discourage worthwhile applicants. "It goes without saying that to inspire others to try a way of life which is still unacceptable to normal society one must in every other way but this be completely normal, above reproach in all things." Suggesting indoor nudity at the first meeting, or requiring applicants to pose for nude pictures as a condition of membership was a sure way to alienate prospective members, and one that backfired on the Sunglades and Quetans clubs.[22]

Although the CSA assured applicants that "you will want to judge them the club organizers just as much as they will be judging you," it was the applicants who were really on trial. First impressions were crucial. People with bad breath and body odor, or over-talkative or boorish, were probably not desirable. This was a social club, after all, and members had to be "good mixers." Nor were applicants with suspect motives desirable: those who wanted pictures, whether of "naked women" to convince a hesitant wife or girlfriend, or of "study subjects showing every part of the male figure," or those who offered self-portraits "sitting on a small bench and showing off a beautiful erection!"[23] Fortunately these questionable applicants usually distinguished themselves by their scintillating verse.

> I was looking true you Book the other day & I Saw you addrest So I taught that I would write you & See if you had Some good pitchers are what have you. I would like fore you to Send me Some naked pitchers. Send me Some Samples of what you got & I will Order Some from you.[24]

Other applicants moved beyond pictorial theory into physical practice by inquiring about "dating," "drinking with girls," and "love making," while a concerned single inquired about the etiquette of erections and the propriety of personal methods for relieving that tension. Still others claimed naturist credentials because they were already into wife swapping or because they had "considerable experience with girls" and were sure they could manage to last "two or three days anyway." Fortunately few of these gentlemen ever showed up for personal interviews.[25]

The real test for the novice came with the first visit to the club. "I can't tell you how many times I've seen people drive up to the gate and then decide to turn around." But here too clubs could take measures to ease the transition. Most do not insist on immediate disrobing for newcomers. Instead, they show prospects around the camp and allow them to become comfortable with the others. After a guided tour first-time visitors are left to themselves, free to join in the activities, to sun by themselves, or to leave if they decide that nudism is not for them after all. But the clubs gamble that most people who have come this far will be tempted by the sun, fresh air, and sports facilities, and will be reassured by the comportment and the camaraderie of the people they meet so that they will indeed join in. The open house experiences of many clubs attest to this.[26]

Ironically, those who were most interested in social nudism and most eager to join were the ones who were most firmly excluded. Single men constituted the largest group of club applicants because men were more likely than women to participate in nude recreation on their own during youth. They tried it, they liked it, and they wanted to participate in a form of nudism that is safe and sociable, so they apply to clubs. And the "decent, sane, and wholesome" clubs turn them away.[27]

Clubs used to shun single applicants because members wanted to maintain some sort of gender balance. In the old-fashioned domestic morality of the 1940s and 1950s nudists argued that "nature fashioned the human animal to be happiest when the sexes are more or less evenly divided." What this meant in practice was that women "do not want to be outnumbered by men," whether the men are single or married. In fact, for many women the "prime pests" were not young single men, but married men trying to get in without their wives and "old bachelors" (middle-aged unmarried men). "The interests of these single men are simply in nude women. . . . Are we women to be admired just like circus animals?" And for their part many married men did not want a surfeit of single men because they "suspect the motives of single men" and assume that everyone was "coming to camp to look at their wives," and they were willing to allow "wife gawking" only on a reciprocal basis.[28]

The other argument that clubs used to justify gender balancing was the focus on family nudism. Social nudism provided a healthy, happy, and safe place to raise children, and nudists could use the presence of children to argue for the decency of nudism on the grounds that as parents they would never expose their children to danger. Even Ray Connett, normally a strong supporter of singles, endorsed this view.

> Remember, nudism is primarily for couples and families. Nudism is tolerated today and has reached its present stage largely because non-nudists and authorities are satisfied that the majority of members are couples and families and that their conduct is above reproach.[29]

Family nudists were not completely heartless towards singles. They had lots of friendly advice to offer as they slammed the door in their faces, most of which can be summarized in the phrase, "come back when you're married." Actually, clubs do not even care if couples are married, as long as they are paired. Wife, mother, sister, daughter—the relationship did not matter so long as the genders were balanced. Unfortunately in some clubs the "logic" of gender balancing led to the expulsion of long-time married members who lost a spouse through death or divorce, and even to quotas on family members' single children as they came of age.[30]

Nudist clubs would seem to be the ideal place for single men to meet single women interested in nudism, but whenever single men raised this point they were shot down. It was up to the single men to go out into conventional society, find a girlfriend, and seduce her into nudism. "There are many girls and ladies who are willing to accompany you if you are a good clean, honest, and well-behaved person." How to convince these ladies of your good intentions? "Next time you swim with a girl ask her if she would mind if you did not use a suit." If she needs more proof, show her nudist magazines and self-portraits. "So, nudist friends across Canada, the best argument for convincing a girl is to show her pictures of yourself in the nude, don't forget that!"[31]

In the meantime single men were encouraged to get out and enjoy the sun, air, and water on their own. "This is Canada where no one need travel more than a dozen miles to find complete outdoor privacy suitable for nudism." Whether on public land with wooded glades, rivers, and deserted lakes or on private land by arrangement with the owner— "most farmers will give you permission to use secluded portions of their wooded land for 'camping'"—nudism was possible for everyone everywhere.

> Nudism alone is better than no nudism at all! Much better to get out of those clothes and be a nudist wherever and whenever you can than to spend a lifetime just thinking and talking about it.[32]

One alternative proposed several times and attempted on occasion was to form a club just for singles—even though Ray Connett himself thought this proposal inappropriate. The most successful singles club was Sunglades in Toronto, which took over a couples group, secured a landed campground, and operated successfully for several years before falling apart in 1953. The most regrettable failure was the International Sunshiners Club in Victoria, organized by two married men in the Vancouver Island Health and Hygiene Club who wanted to keep singles connected with social nudism even if their own club wouldn't accept them. They invited singles to visit camp for two weeks in the summer of 1948. About 130 wrote for information, 30 booked space, and three showed up. The experiment was a failure, although the men who did show up proved to be so sincere and so qualified that they were admitted into the couples club.[33]

A particular point of concern involved teenage boys inspired by reading *Sunbathing for Health* or by their own skinny-dipping experience. In the early days the CSA pointed self-righteously to its constitution with its age-21 rule and shrugged its collective shoulders: "we can do nothing for you." The best that the CSA could offer was to advise boys to show their nudist magazines to their parents and convince them of the propriety of cavorting with a bunch of naked strangers.[34]

In later years some clubs adopted a more open attitude, allowing teens to visit under a variety of pretenses (with parental consent) to "enjoy our clean nude life." The Sunny Trails Club near

Vancouver was particularly active in this regard, accepting a Boy Scout troop that wanted to go swimming nude in the mornings, a teen band that kindly offered to play at club dances free for "experience," and a university students' club that offered clothing-optional recreation to introduce nudism to a wider audience. The "Aborigine Outdoor Club" drew public attention when a concerned parent wrote to columnist Jack Scott about her son's interest in the group. Scott tried to reassure her that "a nudist colony is probably second only to religious retreats as a sanctuary from immorality."

> What the young Aborigines will learn, you see, if their mothers will just stay out of the picture, is that nakedness is natural, pleasant, healthful, attractive, and very often an intelligent way of removing arbitrary tensions between the sexes. ...I have suggested that the mother go along as well, but somehow I don't think she'll take *that* advice.[35]

Supporters of singles argued for the advantages that they could offer clubs. In an oft-quoted phrase, Connett summarized these advantages as "money and muscle." Most single men have jobs and careers like other men, but without the family expenses and obligations, so they could contribute more to the club in cash and work. In some co-op groups, a few singles invested more in the club than all the married members combined, and "they do most of the work."[36]

Today there is another compelling reason for clubs to drop the ban on singles: it is illegal. Several provinces have adopted "human rights" codes that prohibit discrimination along various criteria, including marital status. The assumption behind these codes is that people should be judged on personality and conduct, not on arbitrary superficial aspects. It is also true that the "singles problem" is not exclusively a male problem. Some clubs with strict quotas have even expelled long-time but recently widowed or divorced members, which is another reason why national and international naturist organizations oppose restrictions so vehemently.[37]

Once an organizer established contact with prospective members, the third step in forming a club was to assemble them for a social meeting to discuss past experiences and future expectations, along with practical aspects of club development. These meetings allow members to meet one another in a "normal" social setting and to set up the structure of their club and elect officers. Winter social events (clothed) were important for sustaining interest and for giving prospects "a chance to know us as people first, before having to try us out as nudists at camp." The newly formed group can set out to attract new members who are always necessary for growth in view of the frequent turnover due to loss of interest or change of job.[38]

Unfortunately, nudists have often been hesitant about spreading the word. In the early years of "bootleg nudism," when people were unsure of their legal rights, many nudists were afraid of their own shadow. This self-imposed censorship crimped publicity efforts and hampered growth. Once they have found out about a club and joined, they wanted to keep it the way they found it. They became concerned about opposition, criticism, or ridicule from friends, neighbors, and co-workers. Family secrecy is most problematic, though often even "old-fashioned" relatives can be quite accepting. When Hazel McKague, CSA Secretary in 1951, first told her mother "she was quite shocked," but she realized that "Roy and I would not take the children anyplace that wasn't right." Gradually she met club members at clothed winter functions and learned to like them as people. After two Sundays at camp she joined the club and remained a member until her dying days. "Her last wish was that the club should be represented among the Pall Bearers."[39]

Land for a nudist club can be as small as a back yard or as large as a square mile: whatever is available, appropriate, and affordable. The sine qua non is seclusion; nudists on their own property must not be visible to neighbors or passers-by. Although a lone sunbather might escape detection with a cautionary warning, a mixed group "can expect no mercy from law or publicity."[40]

Several clubs have suffered from peepers, usually teens out on a spying lark or pathetic middle-aged men sitting in the bushes for hours on end to catch a glimpse of free skin when they could be home perusing Playboy. When several intruders are involved managers call the police, who always respond with alacrity. In the 1950s Sun Valley Gardens in Ontario caught a dozen kids with the help of members in cars and on foot, police, two tow trucks, and a surprising number of volunteers. Aside from asserting their own right to privacy, nudists see no reason for "putting on a peep show for every moron who . . . chose to skulk through the bushes like some hungry animal or malevolent spirit." Such incidents demonstrate the need for heavily wooded or otherwise well-screened property. There should be no right of way allowing the public customary transit by land or by water (hikers, fishers, canoeists, hunters). Some members of the Sunny Trails Club learned the hard way that neighbors customarily walked through their woods.[41]

Overflights by air have not been a problem because most aircraft fly high enough not to invade the privacy of groundlings. But there are exceptions, particularly at Lakesun in Ontario which has been buzzed by joy-flying teenagers and by a businessman from Pennsylvania who read about the club, thought it would be a nice place to visit, "borrowed" the company plane, and flew across the border without filing a flight plan to buzz the camp. In both cases the pilots forgot that airplanes have identification numbers under the wings, and so they encountered official receptions upon landing.[42]

Helicopters do present a challenge since they fly at lower altitudes. Ontario Hydro choppers have made appearances over two clubs on routine surveys with different results. In the early 1950s a flight over the secretive Sunglades Club sent members scurrying for clothes and shelter. "The 'copter did not hesitate or back up, so we presume it was legitimately taking the shortest distance between two power projects." But later in the decade a 'copter passed over Otter Lake at Norhaven while two teenage girls were swimming. Being the friendly type they stopped swimming, stood on the beach nude, and waved to the crew. When the men finally noticed the distraction they slammed on the brakes and hovered in mid-air until they realized where they were, waved back, and continued on their way. And at Glen Echo some guests at a nude wedding arrived in the traffic helicopter of a Toronto radio station where one of them worked.[43]

Once a secluded site is located, buying and developing the land forces clubs to structure themselves for the first time. The options were cooperative ownership by the members and proprietary ownership by one member or family. Each type had advantages and disadvantages.

In theory democracy seems attractive: everyone has a voice in the life of the club, everyone participates in the work of the club, and everyone shares in the camaraderie of the club. The problem with democracy in club business is the cacophony of often-uninformed opinion and the partiality to majority sentiment, which leads the minority into silence and eventual departure. If the club members are all newcomers, they may lack the mutual confidence, respect, and trust necessary to persuade them to contribute financially to the future. They may also lack the willingness to do the physical work necessary to develop the campsite, while those who do shoulder the burden resent the freeloaders and the Sunday foremen. "They want a swimming pool, but cannot agree on where it shall be, how it shall be built; what materials to use, how to organise the labor and so on."[44]

Proprietary ownership offered an attractive alternative. Members reluctant to invest in an uncertain future or to work for someone else's benefit could sign over control of the club to one or more members who are willing to buy the land, develop the facilities, and operate the camp for the benefit of the members—who, after all, wanted mainly a place for recreation, not for forced labor—and for whatever profit they can wrest from a seasonal venture with a limited market.[45]

In the 1940s and 1950s Canadian clubs tended to be cooperative (for example, the Van Tans and Sunny Trails in British Columbia, and the Sun Air Freedom Lovers in Ontario) because nudism was a new way of life and nudists were social pioneers. Since the mid-1950s, however, proprietary arrangements have predominated, even where a cooperative social "club" existed but leased land and facilities from a proprietary owner-member (for example, Sunny Chinooks in Alberta and the Toronto Gymnosophical Society).[46]

Regardless of a club's set up, ownership must be registered and zoning permits obtained. The local health department must inspect arrangements for water supply and quality, sewage, and garbage disposal. Police should be notified about the club and invited to visit at any time; this not only ensures a positive working relationship with the police, who may be called on to deal with vandals or snoopers, but creates a good public image: if the police know about it, it must be legal.[47]

Good community relations are an important aspect of club development. Many clubs hold open house days—sometimes nude, sometimes clothed—so that visitors can see what kind of people nudists are and what they do. When Glen Echo invited a "civilian" volleyball team for a match at the club the visitors had "an educational afternoon; and it did more for them than reading about nudism or even being told." Some clubs collect clothing, food, and other necessities for needy families at home and abroad. Others have made their camp facilities available to the community for various activities.

> Each year we entertain various members of the village, classes from our high school, at camp, with hot dog roasts, feeds, and picnics. All know they are being entertained at a nudist camp. The only criticism we have heard about the parties is that we do not have them often enough.[48]

Once a club is established, what do nudists do? Nudity itself is not the main attraction, but what else is there? In the early days facilities were simple. People were glad just to have a secure place for sunbathing, so anything else was a welcome addition. Besides, most early clubs were cooperative, and so everyone had to spend time clearing the land, building a clubhouse, and setting up their own cabins, tents, or trailers. But eventually the heavy work was finished, and members set about providing amenities. The most basic feature of every club was some kind of swimming hole—and most of the early ones were literally "mudholes" created by damming a river or dredging out a spring, although a few lucky clubs had natural ponds or even lakes. Basic hygienic facilities were next: cold showers and outdoor privies. A little later, clubs might add a grass court for volleyball and badminton, and pitching courts for horseshoes. The clubhouse itself might serve to accommodate table tennis and board games on rainy days. And the children needed playground equipment: swings, slides, teeter totters, monkey bars, and merry-go-rounds.[49]

In the 1960s and 1970s clubs got larger and offered a greater variety of facilities and activities. Besides ensuring better campground basics—hot showers, indoor flush toilets (segregated, unlike the showers), and full utility hook-ups for campers, trailers, and Recreational Vehicles—most clubs now offered concrete or vinyl in-ground swimming pools, saunas, and whirlpools or hot tubs. The range of games also expanded. Most clubs now offered badminton, shuffleboard, tennis, mini-golf, softball, miniten, and petanque, in addition to the ubiquitous volleyball. In the 1970s several clubs expanded their clubhouses or built new ones to provide heated indoor swimming pools for year-round nudism. And for rainy days card and board games, darts, table tennis, billiards, and video games were available. Clubs that stay open all year round not only offer cozy indoor swimming but frosty outdoor activity as well: cross-country skiing, snowmobiles, tobogganing, and ice skating are all popular among these polar bares. Other popular events are the interclub competitions in a variety of summer games and sports, primarily volleyball tournaments played according to official Volleyball Association rules with official referees and sometimes with outside teams that agree to play "in uniform" against nudist teams (which face their own competition in the Nude Volleyball Superbowl at White Thorn Lodge in Pennsylvania, where the Glen Echo and Richard Brunet clubs excel). And for the seriously adventurous types a B.C. group offered nude bungee jumping.[50]

Social events also take place at the typical club all year. Besides the special games, tournaments, and "olympics" in the summer, clubs hold dances and parties on weekends summer and winter. The dances are clothed because "we don't want to have to throw a bucket of cold water on a couple dancing," and are held at the drop of a thematic hat: Valentine's, Easter, Greaser Fifties, Westerns, Hawaiian, Pyjamas, Togas, Thanksgiving, Halloween, Christmas, New Year's. There are movie nights for adults (nudist videos on other clubs for armchair or prospective travellers), for children (cartoons), and for families ("where *Free Willy* is sure to be the summer smash"). And there is always the ubiquitous barbecue.

> There beside the warm camp fire-side
> By the pool of shining water
> There they roasted in the fire flame
> Weiners, meaty, brown and tasty.
> Weiners scorched upon the outside
> Burnt and flaming on the skinside
> Cold and raw upon the inside.
> None the less with skin side inside
> Rolls all crusty on the outside
> Was the sacrificial weiner
> Eaten as a sign of friendship.[51]

CHAPTER THREE

Evergreen Tans

The first organized group of social nudists in British Columbia gathered in the 1930s at a summer camp in Port Alberni on the West Coast of Vancouver Island. Later, Captain Dick Parritt made available a private yacht accommodating a dozen passengers for a four hour cruise through the Alberni Inlet and Barkley Sound (now part of Pacific Rim National Park). The Alberni group organized officially in 1952 in affiliation with the Canadian Sunbathing Association. The new group leader, Trevor, acquired several islands in Sproat Lake, making for "a nudist paradise, completely alone."[1]

Nudist activity on the Island naturally centered in Victoria, which at times had more clubs than members. In the early 1940s two residents came in contact through articles in Canadian and American magazines. The first was Jim Sewell, who supported various clubs, including the Sun-Air-Freedom-Lovers in Ontario. In 1942 he proposed to form the Victoria Sunair Club and to make available a portion of his land for the camp, to be called Sunacres. But then another local nudist, Mex Starkey, appeared on the scene. At first Sewell was "looking forward to some good nudist outings with him," but gradually their personalities clashed to the point where cooperation became difficult, if not impossible.[2]

Starkey, originally from Ontario, also acquired land in the mountains, 85 acres on the Koksilah River, which during the mid-1940s became home for the Vancouver Island Health and Hygiene Club. At first the club was simply a group of contacts whom Mex and his wife Alice invited to meet on their land. In 1949, at the instigation of the recently formed Canadian Sunbathing

Association, they decided to organize. By this time family matters affecting both organizers, as well as personal tensions between them, led the CSA to co-opt another family, the Greens, to assume responsibility for the Victoria club. In February about a dozen people attended the first meeting, including the Greens, Starkey, and Joan Skipper, later a leading figure in the Van Tan Club, the CSA, and the WCSA. Jim and Nancy, a local couple, allowed the group to use part of their in-town land for sunbathing, while Mex invited the group to his up-country location for more extensive recreation. Yet another small group—the Victoria People—operated separately in Royal Oak. None the less, the lack of unity was counterproductive. By the end of 1949 the Greens had to admit that "to all intents and purposes the club doesn't exist," and they resolved to "get those nudists here, who are reasonably compatible, together" and to try to hold on until a new club could start over.[3]

In 1951 Albert Young set out to organize single "lovers of naked sunbathing, swimming and outdoor sport." Young was a member of the CSA and arranged membership for other singles during the open house days at the Van Tan and Border Tan clubs. He proposed to form a group for single men and women, using secluded places around Victoria. In 1952 George Luff joined him. Together they started investigating sites for summer use, including Mex Starkey's land. In 1953 the group acquired land of its own and formally organized as the Pac Sun Club.[4]

Although Pac Sun built on the singles group foundation laid by Young and Luff, it operated as "an up and coming mixed group club." The Pac Suns acquired 192 acres just off the Malahat Highway twenty miles north of Victoria. By 1955 the club comprised fifteen members, including three families and three single women, and advertised in Sunny Trails. But that same year the Sooke Community Association voted against granting nudists access to a public swimming area—the Pemberton pool—and the club relocated to a rented site, three hundred acres in the Metochsin area. This location proved unsuitable to the members (as did one of the founders), and so the majority left Metochsin and started over once again, reverting to the original group function as a social club for singles.[5]

The rest remained on the land temporarily but reorganized and renamed themselves as Sol Sante. In 1956 Sol Sante acquired 250 acres near Shawnigan Lake, about 30 miles from Victoria. The land included a private spring-fed lake (Little Shawnigan) for swimming, fishing, and boating, fields for volleyball and badminton, and a farmhouse with electricity and running water, which provided a ready-made clubhouse. Sol Sante's most distinctive feature is a totem pole carved by a club member and mounted beside the lake. The figures on the totem represent the elements, the sun, humanity, children, wildlife, and the lake itself.[6]

Sol Sante officially opened its gates on the first weekend of June 1956, when CSA officials and members from other BC clubs journeyed to Cobble Hill to present the club with its CSA/ASA charter. All were sufficiently impressed with the new club to select it as the site of the 1957 CSA-West convention.[7]

The teething years of the Sol Sante Club were more difficult than for most clubs as it had to face three serious crises. In 1957 personality and policy conflicts with the club president led several members to quit and to file complaints, which the CSA temporarily resolved.[8] Second, the club now had to complete the purchase of its land and develope facilities and cabins, which they accomplished by selling off a section of property and by allowing members to buy their own campsites. Third, the club revoked camera rights for its photographer for taking pictures of members without approval and publishing them in nudist magazines without consent. His replacement promised "many fine photographs of this club with more of the fairer sex being photographed."[9]

Some of the disgruntled members who left Sol Sante in 1958 formed a new group—the Victoria Sunbathing Club—with the former Sol Sante president as their leader. They acquired nine acres of land back in the Metochsin area. The new club found a unique public relations gambit when members offered their services to the Victoria Art Gallery, which had reported difficulty finding nude models for art classes. But such gestures could not finance club development of the club, and in 1960 members voted to rejoin Sol Sante, which appeared to have resolved its internal troubles.[10]

During the 1960s Sol Sante hosted several conventions, including the ASA national convention in 1965 that nearly bankrupted the club. Attendance at a rustic camp at the far end of North America appealed to only about 300 ASA members, and the low attendance did not compensate the club for the effort and expense members invested into developing the club. And, like many other clubs in the 1960s, Sol Sante went through major changes in membership and attitude. A younger, Canadian-born generation and a newer immigrant membership had little experience with, or tolerance for, restrictive Canadian regulations on alcohol, and saw no reason why their recreational clubs should uphold the ASA's rigid policy towards the normal social activity of moderate drinking— particularly when several empty liquor bottles were discovered in the sleeping quarters of ASA delegates after the convention. These developments persuaded the club to vote for a trial separation from the ASA, which was confirmed in 1967 when Sol Sante became one of several clubs to quit the ASA after hosting a national convention. For a number of years its only contact with the outside world would be its annual participation in the Labor Day festivities at Sunny Trails, also an ASA dropout. But more recently the club has changed its policy and welcomes visitors to its beautiful corner of Canada.[11]

When Sol Sante voted to quit the WCSA/ASA, some dissidents left to form the Nanaimo Tans, under Charlie Roy, later president of the WCSA. On 18 acres of wooded, rocky land the club set up an in-ground pool, sauna, and clubhouse; courts for volleyball, badminton, and miniten; and a merry-go-round for kids. In 1970, when the club hosted its first WCSA convention, it had about fifty members. The following year the club hosted a wedding between two members; the bride and groom wore "an even coat of tan." Then the club faced "a trying time . . . on a legal battle" concerning title to their land. Although the dispute was settled favorably, the club lost many members while its future seemed uncertain.[12]

As the fortunes of the Nanaimo Tans waned, ASA faithful moved down-island once again to form Arbutus Park, a travel club based in the homes of its members, including the president's home with indoor pool and hot tub. Members visited nearby landed clubs in BC and the U.S. Northwest. Up-island the Tsolumaires briefly tried to carry on the Nanaimo Tans tradition in Courtenay before dissolving in 1973.[13]

The real future of BC nudism lay on the lower mainland. In 1939 Edward Lansdowne placed a short "Personals" ad in the *Vancouver Province*: "Member of N.S.A.A. wishes to form similar club here." To faithful readers of *Health & Efficiency*, the British nudist magazine, these "magic initials" stood for the National Sun and Air Association. A handful of men (wives were not encouraged to attend this first meeting) gathered to compare notes on local sunbathing experiences and to discuss forming a club in Vancouver. Besides Lansdowne, attendees included Ray Connett (later secretary of the Van Tans before leaving to form his own Sunny Trails Club), Ronald Walker (who founded the Border Tans), and Hardy and Lenore Kaye (the driving force in the early Van Tans). He was English, she Australian; both were en route from a vacation in England—where they had just experienced nudism for the first time at the Arcadians club—back to Australia when they got stranded in Canada at the outbreak of war.[14]

During the next few weeks and months the group went to "'look for land.' That was our excuse for a number of outings." One favored spot was an island in the Alouette River near Coquitlam, which they visited several times (now with the wives). Meanwhile Ron checked real estate listings and Alisdair, a civil servant in Victoria, checked government records for surveyed lots available in the North Vancouver area, and this is how the Van Tan Club (named by Stella Walker) came to roost on Grouse Mountain. Alisdair bought some land part way up the mountain and took the others to inspect it. One look around—at the "loveliest panoramic view" of Vancouver 1,500 feet below, the Fraser River valley, Mt Baker, the Georgia Strait, and the mountains of Vancouver Island and the Olympic Peninsula in the distance—and everyone was hooked: "you just felt like gods on Olympus."[15]

The war put the club in hiatus for several years. Some of the men, like Ray Connett, went off to Europe. For the rest, wartime shortages and controls limited their ability to develop the campsite. But the war ended, and the Van Tans shifted back into gear. In 1947 the club settled its land title. When members registered the title transfer the District Commissioner informed them that adjacent lots were also available, and so the club expanded to embrace four acres owned and three acres leased. When the Van Tans incorporated, their lawyer assured them that "the purposes of the club can be so generalized as to attract no attention."[16]

By this time the Kayes had resigned their positions in the club and nominated Ray Connett as club secretary, which post he held until 1948. Connett brought a commitment to publicity as a means of growth for the club and for nudism in general. He believed that a newsletter "will build your club faster than any other way" and used the *Van Tan Call* to inform members of activities, to coordinate work schedules, and to arrange rides for members without cars. The *Call* would have an on-again, off-again existence over the years, but it remains one of the more popular club newsletters in Canada.[17]

Publicity is vital for any club that wants to grow and prosper, but the Van Tans preferred "a policy of careful secrecy." In 1946 Connett, as "one or two of the more progressive members—shall we even call them 'radicals',” persuaded the club to endorse brief notices to the newspapers regarding nudist clubs in the States visited by "local nudists." Panic ensued when the papers wanted to learn more about these "local nudists," and one or two members quit and never returned. But when nothing bad happened, the club got bolder, giving out press releases left and right and inviting reporters to visit the club. "We have found that newspapers are reliable businesses and that they can be trusted to cooperate if given some hope of news, which is their business."[18]

This forthright approach paid off in 1952 when a story appeared in the *Vancouver Sun* claiming that a neighbor living on Grouse Mountain had complained about "Black Bears, Bare Whites on North Shore Highway." Van Tan representatives immediately contacted the Sun and the RCMP, and learned that the woman had indeed filed a complaint—against teenagers drinking and necking on the road at night. She never mentioned "bare whites on the highway," she just wanted city hall to put in street lights to keep people off her road and mentioned everything and everyone she had ever heard of to get attention.[19]

During the war the club had adopted a "no singles" policy, but Connett and the Kayes persuaded members to reconsider. In 1947 the Van Tans approved a quota of five single men for each three single women. Several pending applications were approved, "and none has ever given the slightest cause for offense"; some were even elected to club office. Eventually the club dropped its quota completely because by the end of the decade the club was "so near on the rocks" that "we needed money—and we needed workers."[20]

One reason for the workers was the perennial damage the club suffered. Like many isolated developments in the mountains of B.C., the Van Tan Club often fell victim to vandals. At first the break-ins were merely disturbing, as the perpetrators "neatly and expertly pried off" the lock on the clubhouse, took nothing, and "closed the door behind them." A bigger and better lock failed to deter the intruders, who continued to "leave everything unharmed, even swept the floor last week." Soon the visitors made themselves more at home: "the chairs were left in a cozy circle around the stove, a can of beans was gone and all the coffee." Then the games ceased and the vandals got down to business, tossing beds over the mountain, doing serious damage to the clubhouse, and leaving behind a threatening note which the club passed on to the police. But the police could not patrol all the time, so the club decided to hire a resident caretaker. Norman became a fixture during the early 1950s, and helped deter unwanted visitors (and even some wanted ones, if they lacked proper identification), but one day someone noticed a bottle in the trash, and Norman was asked to leave. The vandals promptly returned and became a regular feature of the winter months. At times the recurrent damage was so extensive that the club was able to negotiate a reduction in their property tax assessment.[21]

At the end of the war membership was barely two dozen adults, attendance was sparse, and little work was being done. The future looked bleak. Improvements were imperative, but they cost money, and the club had a hard enough time repaying $150 for their land. In 1947 Roy McKague, newly arrived from Ontario, brought with him a shareholding plan to finance payments and improvements based on the Sun-Air model. Members would contribute a set amount over and above regular annual dues, which would entitle them to share in the ownership of the club and to be eligible for election to club office. The amount collected would be earmarked for major development projects that could not be financed otherwise. Although club members modified this plan to allow everyone to contribute, not simply "charter members," and also voted to continue their group work program, the new policy succeeded in raising badly needed funds for key projects.[22]

Two developments topped the agenda for 1948: relocating the clubhouse closer to the gate and revamping the swimming pool. As it happened the two projects meshed more closely than anticipated, because the bulldozer that came in to level the site for the new clubhouse destroyed the club gate and also "ripped out the pitiful little pool" created the previous year, when the Van Tans hosted their first Open House for nearby club members. When Connett and his singles brigade dug into the ground where the old clubhouse had been they found a natural rock bottom with a gentle slope, perfectly suited for a bigger and better pool. It took a while to excavate a hole large enough for a 25-by-40 foot pool, but one fine day in June 1952 forty members, under the direction of "Tiny" MacDonald (for whom the pool was named after his death in 1995) formed a continuous relay of water buckets to mix and pour the cement walls for the new pool, which was then filled with water stored behind the club's own dam (itself an occasional target of vandals). This pool lasted more than thirty-five years, with only one major resurfacing in the late sixties, before the club installed a new vinyl liner in 1988. Over the years the pool was joined by volleyball and shuffleboard courts, a sauna, and a wading pool for the children.[23]

Another postwar innovation were the indoor winter meetings which kept members in touch. At first these were purely social gatherings in members' homes. But in 1947 the club decided to rent the school gymnasium in nearby Lynn Valley for dances and volleyball games. In later years the Van Tans rented the Hendry Community Hall for winter dances that were eagerly anticipated by the custodian: "he said that in all the years he had cared for Hendry Hall he had never met such a well mannered group as the Van Tan Club." More recently, the club has rented the William Griffin pool for monthly swim nights during the winter, after several years of renting saunas.[24]

The more the club expanded in facilities and in members, the more willing it was to extend its publicity. Starting in 1947 it hosted open house days for members of nearby clubs, and—after a bitter internal debate—for CSA members. In 1954, with the new clubhouse and swimming pool in place, the Van Tans held their first Open House for the general public, which has become an annual event.[25] On May 24, 1970, "a glorious warm sunny day," the Van Tans hosted their first nude open house. This, too, became an annual event, culminating in the 1989 Open House on June 4, when the Van Tans celebrated their golden anniversary with full media coverage—the first Canadian club to reach this milestone.[26]

The Border Tan Club was formed on 21 January 1948 by some Van Tan members residing in the Lower Fraser Valley who were weary of the long drive to North Vancouver and tired of paying bridge tolls. By April the group found land in Langley which the owner leased to the club for one dollar a year and first option to buy. The campground was named Sunnybrook, and the newsletter was called the Border Tan Echo. In its first summer the club attracted twenty-one members.[27]

The club received more than its share of unwanted attention. Snoopers who threatened to "run the nudists out" were a temporary nuisance until the police threatened to run the snoopers out. More vocal opposition came from members of a religious sect who demanded that authorities act "to ban this evil influence which was attracting their teen-age sons to snooping about the bushes." Club members took to the offensive by writing letters to the press and to the municipal council. Police were invited to inspect the camp, and reported on the high moral character of the members. The Border Tans quickly became an accepted part of the community and the club was listed prominently in newspaper reports as "the nudist colony which attracts sunbathers from both sides of the International border to Langley's banana belt."[28]

Sunnybrook Park occupied six acres in a sheltered valley surrounding a stream. Over time, members built or installed a clubhouse, a swimming pool, a wading pool, volleyball courts, and a children's playground with swings and teeter-totters. During winter they rented a sauna for monthly get-togethers. Although Border Tans was a relatively small club it was actively involved in CSA affairs. In its short history it hosted three CSA conventions which attracted hundreds of visitors. The club inaugurated the practice of holding open house days for the general public, although the first occasion, in 1952, was hampered by poor weather. After several changes of ownership, the club was sold to the Boy Scouts in 1956.[29]

Two other small clubs operated in the lower mainland around this time. In 1950 Ray Connett, chafing at the conservatism of the Van Tan Club and anxious to show Canadians how to organize nudism properly, created a "really novel enterprise"—a social club designed to provide indoor activities during the winter. The new group was called the Health and Sun Society (HASS), after the CSA rejected Connett's bid for the name Sunny Trails, which it used for its own magazine, edited by Connett.[30]

In its first months HASS rented a steam bath and offered sauna and sunlamps for members and guests. Connett also hosted soirées in his home, with ping pong, darts, cards, and games. By summer 1950 he was able to provide outdoor sunning in the half-acre of enclosed back yard adjoining his home on Sea Island. Although the HASS experiment did not last very long, it gave Connett the experience and encouragement he needed to form the highly successful Sunny Trails Club in 1952.[31]

The other small club was Tebbutt Nature Park in Port Kells, about 20 miles southeast of Vancouver. The owner made his private ten-acre rustic site available for people who sought the simple enjoyment of sun, fresh air, and rest in the great outdoors. Although the park had only sun, air, and trees, the private grounds adjoined Port Kells public park, which had a swimming pool. But the limited facilities at Tebbutts Park, at a time when the Van Tans, Border Tans, and Sunny Trails were all developing rapidly, along with the advanced age of the owners, made Tebbutts a short-lived but well-regarded club.[32]

The Sunny Trails Club originated in 1952, when Ray Connett accepted a chance invitation to visit a farm in Surrey. Though a longtime member of the Van Tan Club, he had his own vision of what a nudist club should be. For years he had criticized the Van Tans for their secrecy. Inspired by the success that American clubs had with publicity, he believed the time was ripe for similar action in Canada. Besides, he was tired of sitting in the rain on Grouse Mountain and watching the sun shining in Surrey.[33]

When a Surrey farmer waiting in the post office where Connett worked overheard him tell another customer about his desire for land suitable for a nature park, and the farmer happened to have land available, Ray's interest was aroused. After doing some preliminary clearing on the land during the summer, Connett invited CSA and local club members to visit the site on Labor Day. They found twenty secluded acres of woodland with two babbling brooks, only 20 miles from downtown Vancouver. They immediately accepted a long-term lease with option to buy. A little later they learned that the neighbor who owned a back road leading into their camp was anxious to sell his land also, and so Sunny

Trails became owner of 22 acres of land in addition to the 20 that it leased, making it the second-largest camp in Canada, after Norhaven in Ontario.[34]

From the start Connett saw Sunny Trails more as an experiment than as an enterprise. The club would embody ideas that he had been preaching for years. As he modestly wrote in 1953, "the Sunny Trails Club is backed by the finances of a group of nudists who are probably the most advanced thinkers in the movement today. Many of the outstanding accomplishments of the past have come through their efforts." He and his associates proposed, first, to open the club to all applicants of good character without discrimination or quotas against single men (although this policy changed very quickly) and, second, to implement an "open forthright publicity policy" to promote nudism and preempt opposition.[35]

The need for "damage control" public relations became apparent sooner than expected. During the first winter several members frequently spent weekends working at camp to get it ready for the formal opening, in the spring of 1953. On one of these occasions some local children who were walking in the woods observed the nudists and reported them. The Parent-Teacher Association took the news in stride. One woman remarked to a male colleague that she would join the club if he would. Nevertheless, it was obvious to Ray Connett that public opposition would be dangerous, and that the best defense was a good PR offense. He met with the RCMP, City Hall, the Chamber of Commerce, and the school to explain the club and nudism. When the Municipal Council debated the issue it endorsed Sunny Trails as "legal and above board."[36]

In summer of 1953 Sunny Trails inaugurated its "forthright" publicity plan by inviting the public to visit the camp on a weekend when members would be dressed. On Saturday, 18 July, some 250 local residents were greeted by 125 nudists, including many from other B.C. and U.S. clubs (though not from the Border Tans, who boycotted the new club). The next day clergy and local officials toured the camp while members were in uniform to witness the formal granting of a CSA charter to the club. Newspaper and radio reporters covered the event, and CBC radio presented a nationwide broadcast. As a promotional event, it was an unqualified success.[37]

Throughout the 1950s Sunny Trails went from one publicity triumph to another. In 1954 the open house on "Charter Weekend" was well-advertised, and this time town councillors, members of clergy, and representatives of municipal service organizations attended in force. On Saturday 250 people toured the grounds while members remained dressed. On Sunday two dozen dignitaries attended with the nudists nude and witnessed a royal family contest as part of the CSA national convention. All the officials present had nothing but praise for the club. And two PTA representatives, who spent most of their time at camp "ardently contemplating the heavens," none the less conceded that Sunny Trails had "a very nice location." Only Jean Howarth, a reporter for the *Vancouver Province*, considered nudism "a deviation from the healthy norm." But club members took her remarks in stride, noting that "she couldn't see the women for looking at the men!" Howarth herself conceded that "I shall never attend a meeting again, without fancying the chairman in his birthday suit."[38]

The crowning achievement of Sunny Trails publicity was the nude open house in 1959. When the event took place, on Sunday, 16 August 1959, the response was overwhelming: 2,327 adults came, some with their children. Couples, families, and single women were admitted after signing a statement that they would not be offended by nudity, and—as the *Vancouver Sun* reported—"everybody approved. Some came out of curiosity, others to gawk or ridicule. But they all left impressed."[39] There was the usual amount of media coverage for a Sunny Trails event, and in addition the CBC-TV affiliate CBUT filmed the event and broadcast it after the early evening news. But the open house, though an unqualified success, was clearly a one-shot phenomenon; a repeat the following year drew only a few hundred visitors.[40]

Beneath the glitter and glamor of all this public relations hype the club grew steadily, quickly topping the 100 member mark. Many of these early members were single men whom Connett recruited because they had three things that a growing club need-ed: time, money, and stamina. All members were subjected to his "unusual work policy," which required them to put in time and effort every weekend on various development projects, from clear-ing land through excavating the swimming pool—"Walker Lake"—to building the clubhouse. In their spare time they were supposed to work on their own campsites, particularly the cabins that would dot the ridge later known as Snob Hill.[41]

Connett felt a justifiable but somewhat overstated pride in this accomplishment.

> A brave new club has formed in Canada, a club with a future which could not be more brilliant, which could not have made more progress since its inception, had a star risen above it to herald its beginning.[42]

But pride goes before the fall, and so it was at Sunny Trails. Connett thought that the work program was a constructive way to develop the club quickly with limited resources and believed that "the work is not carried to extremes." Members begged to differ, especially in reaction to his "grandiose" plans of the mid-1950s for a "great new complex" including a clubhouse, dance hall, restaurant, covered volleyball court, "and half a dozen other things. Ray was really dreaming on this one." In 1955 the members staged a revolt against their "one-man club," the work brigades with their "concen-tration camp" atmosphere, and Ray's personal "dictatorship."[43]

Connett survived this inquisition, which reflected the tensions of running a cooperative club that needed development but cher-ished individual freedom. In 1957 the club offered the Connetts positions as paid managers. But by this time Ray was frustrated in his post office job, where he was demoted because of his "outside activities," and where it became obvious that his high-profile nud-ist activity precluded further promotion; frustrated with the club and with the CSA, which split apart in 1956; and frustrated with in

BC rain when sunny California, which the Connetts visited in early 1957, beckoned with year-round sunshine and nudism. In October they loaded up their trailer and moved to Olive Dell. Later he founded Glen Eden in Corona, California. The Connetts remained Life Members of Sunny Trails, despite one board's mean-spirited attempt to revoke the honor in the early 1970s. Ray and Mildred died at Glen Eden in 1997.[44]

The true love of Sunny Trails members has always been politics. From day 1, infighting, bickering, quarrelling, and backstabbing have been facts of club life; in the words of the club historian, "we commit suicide regularly." The main bone of contention has concerned land and land financing. When Sunny Trails started in 1952, members arranged to lease 20 acres and to buy another. Part of the leasing arrangement gave the owner the right to offer the land for sale, and in 1959 he put up 15 acres for sale, keeping the rest for his retirement home. The club agreed to buy the land for $3,500 down and $100 per month, and set up a Land Purchase Fund, based on compulsory loans to the club from each member, which replaced the earlier shareholding arrangement.[45]

Two years later the owner, anxious for payment, offered to sell out for $12,000. The board felt unable to accept this price, but one member, Winnie, negotiated a private arrangement to acquire the greement of sale, and thereby "bought the Club right out from under the members' noses." She and her husband started receiving the $100 per month which the club was pledged to pay.[46]

At the same time members became increasingly frustrated by the number of major projects—pool, volleyball court, toilets, well, power lines—which "seem to have been tailored to fit an opium inspired pipedream of a grandiose nudist empire," and never seemed to get completed, thereby creating a "perpetual construction camp presided over by a handful of frustrated empire builders." The tense atmosphere undermined morale throughout 1961 and laid the foundation for a dramatic coup d'etat in 1962.[47]

In December 1961 the soon-to-be-president, Herman, drafted

an "Emergency Program" to cope with the financial crisis and members' dissatisfaction with the "unhappy atmosphere" in the club. Other members who shared these sentiments set up the Sunny Trails Reform Committee—an "informal, voluntary group which has formed in response to the potentially disastrous situation confronting our club"—and issued a circular on 12 January 1962, warning members that "your sunbathing club is in imminent danger of collapse. Unless drastic corrective action is taken immediately, the club is unlikely to survive the year."[48]

The stage was set for yet another "kerfuffle." As the club historian wrote later, "the day of the big meeting came upon an unsuspecting board. We were caught with our pants down if any one ever was." The Reform Committee had planned well, and arrived armed with a clear-cut strategy: election of a neutral chairman pro tem, a vote of non-confidence in the board, and election of a new board to cope with the emergency. A flood of discussion ensued about projects and finances, including the perennial agreement of sale issue. After considerable debate the president resigned, followed by other members of the board, and an emergency board was elected in its place. Two former board members were kept on "so there could be a form of continuity." The whole coup lasted three and one-half hours. Again quoting the club historian, "it was one of the most dramatic things to be part of. I just had to admire Bob . . . as he stood there with an iron will and engineered one of the slickest political cons I'll ever probably see."[49]

The first actions of the new board were to reconsider the ASA convention scheduled for summer 1962 at Sunny Trails, and to negotiate a suspension of affiliation with the ASA and the WCSA until the club could put its financial house in order. The breach would last nearly twenty years.[50] The club's financial predicament took awhile longer to sort out. Not until January 1963 did the new board present a "package plan" for refinancing the debt by raising dues and enforcing payment. The plan was approved by a nearly unanimous vote. When the Greater Vancouver Regional Development Authority expropriated the club land in 1970 for future parkland, the club paid off the balance owing to Peter, and also bought out the cabin owners on Snob Hill.[51]

The coup of 1962 meant more than a restructuring of club finances. At the same time the board announced its five year plan for major construction projects on the sauna, well, pool, restrooms, and clubhouse. Together with these physical changes came dramatic socio-cultural changes which amounted to a "revolution . . . in the realm of ideas and personal freedom." Actually, club members began to question traditional rituals such as open house days and nudist mother contests as soon as Ray and Mildred left for California.[52]

After Sunny Trails disaffiliated from the ASA it dropped many ASA strictures on personal conduct. It abolished the "ridiculous" rules against touching, drinking, and "colorful language." These changes added up to a "new nudist look." The club replaced compulsory nudity with a clothing-optional policy, requiring nudity only in the pool, sauna, and hot tub. Though intended as liberating innovations, these changes "OPENED THE DOORS" to more serious—and more questionable—behavior. In 1969 the club split over the issue of "touchy-feely" sessions. Sympathizers argued that the club should make room for a "non-verbal communications seminar" and become a "progressive" club which would "grow and expand with the times," while opponents denigrated the "crazy sessions" and "Love-Ins." Many traditionalists broke away to form the Meadowbrook Club, which Sunny Trails regarded as "an affront to our efforts."[53]

In 1968 the Vancouver-Fraser Park Board announced plans to develop a major park and zoo in Surrey on land fronting the Trans-Canada Highway. In 1970 it appropriated Sunny Trails and became the proud owner of a nudist club. The terms of sale allowed the club to remain on the Surrey property with a renewable lease until it located and developed another site. In September the club bought 30 acres in south Surrey, not far from the U.S. border. Unfortunately the Eighth Avenue property, as rural land, was zoned for agricultural use. When the club petitioned for rezoning, the municipal council refused, partly because of the "amount of naked flesh" visible to neighbors. The club met this defeat with a declaration that it would keep its land even if it had to develop it agriculturally—thus thwarting the "ambitious vote-conscious" mayor of Surrey, Bill Vander Zalm, who confessed that "I thought if their application failed they'd just go away."[54]

Since development at Eighth Avenue was blocked, the club decided to channel its development budget into removable improvements on the existing property, including an in-ground pool, sauna, hot tub, snack bar, and games room. Fiscal restraint during the 1970s hindered development of Tynehead Park, which gave the club an indefinite stay of execution.[55]

When it became clear that the Eighth Avenue property would never be acceptable to members or neighbors, the club resumed its search for a new home. After years of looking and inspecting, it found a trailer park at Lake Errock, east of Mission in the Fraser Valley, which boasted "a panoramic view of some of the most beautiful mountains in British Columbia." (The area was already home to a rustic vacation camp, Mountain Haven, started in 1988 by a former Sunny Trails president.) The club purchased the property, which was zoned for recreational/commercial use, and sold the Eighth Avenue property in the summer of 1988. In 1992 the club made the move to its new home in time to celebrate its fortieth anniversary, and in 1994 it hosted a WCSA convention for the first time in more than three decades.[56]

The Meadowbrook Sun Club was formed in April 1963 by a dozen former Sunny Trails members dissatisfied with the new policies inaugurated at that club in the early sixties, particularly the relaxation of time-honored ASA rules regarding touching, drinking, and swearing. The new club also affirmed its commitment to nudity at a time when Sunny Trails switched to clothing-optional status. Meadowbrook immediately applied for ASA/WCSA membership.[57]

One member of the new group arranged to buy land in Surrey,

which he leased to the club. Committees were made responsible for social activities and for suggesting developments to the grounds. But during the first season, as membership rose to thirty, it became evident that the club needed a new structure in order to develop more facilities, especially a proper swimming pool. At the general meeting in October 1963 the landowner proposed to take over the club completely so as to accelerate development. He promised to install a sauna and swimming pool in time for the 1964 season. On this basis the club accepted the proprietary arrangement, and also submitted a bid to host the 1964 WCSA convention.[58]

Despite this initial burst of enthusiasm, problems arose between the club and the owner; "most of us couldn't put up with him any longer." From October 1965 until May 1966 the club had no campground, and membership fell off sharply. Then, in April 1966, a group of members raised a loan and bought a new site in Aldergrove—five acres of land, an old log house that became a temporary clubhouse, and a well. Members quickly added a pond for the kids and volleyball, badminton, and horseshoes for the adults. While waiting for their in-ground pool to be completed they made use of the Olympic Swim Center in Whalley. By 1968, when Meadowbrook again hosted the WCSA convention, membership had climbed back up to fifty adults with thirty children, and the club started to expand its facilities again.[59]

All this development cost money—more than the club had, as ambitions outran assets—and also required work, which exceeded members' initiative. The response was two-fold: a consortium of members formed the Nu-Deal company to assume the club's assets, liabilities, and operating expenses, while a "strong public relations program" set out to attract new members.[60]

In September 1969 Meadowbrook organized a "Nude Fun Fair" open to the public and to visitors from other clubs. They sold tickets for sports and games and for the opportunity to throw wet "sock it to me" sponges at the camp manager, who was a big "Laugh-In" fan. More than 200 people attended, and only six declined to get in uniform. Fun fairs were held for several years afterwards. In 1970 Meadowbrook held its first open house. Visitors were allowed in while members were dressed; they toured the grounds and watched the ASA promotional film, "The Take-Off." In 1972 the club presented the nudist play "Barely Proper."[61]

The most successful—and controversial—publicity campaign was the Miss Nude Pacific Northwest competition in 1972. The contest was affiliated with the Miss Nude World competition at the Four Seasons club in Ontario. The first time around five contestants faced five judges, who chose Lorraine from the Lake Associates Club near Seattle. Sunny Trails sponsored two contestants, one of whom placed third. The STC newsletter revealed lingering feelings towards Meadowbrook when the editor gloated because the Meadowbrook contestants had dropped out because of "tan problems," and remarked on the evening's entertainment featuring "booze" (at a club that had quit Sunny Trails because of its liberal policy on alcohol) and dancing to the "melancholy *stains* of the Meadowlarks." But Meadowbrook got more favorable coverage on CBC news and local cable TV. Six newspapers also reported on the contest, which was attended by 150 non-nudists.[62]

In 1973 the club repeated the contest and the winner; Lorraine again defeated her competition, which included two Meadowbrook entries who placed second and third. By this time some club members became obsessed with winning. In 1974 they entered professional strippers as their official contestants (one of whom nearly had to drop out when she admitted that she had "almost paid" her membership dues, since the contest was supposed to be open only to bona fide nudists). Although club members and legitimate contestants complained, the board confirmed Patty Knight, a "professional dancer and model," as the contest winner. A reporter noted that Patty would face "likely stiffer competition" at the Miss Nude World contest.[63]

Unknown to all, this contest marked the beginning of the end for Meadowbrook. Several disgruntled members left to form the Hyperion Club, while the board entrenched itself firmly. Then other members started to raise the standard issue for clubs in financial trouble: cutting affiliation with the ASA. In February 1975 members overwhelmingly voted to stay with ASA/WCSA; a year later the club did vote to leave, by 18 to 11. Questions were raised about how many members had received notice of the meeting, and about the voting procedure, but the result stood, and the board gave official notice to the ASA in 1976. The board then set out to purge several longtime members for various petty personal and political reasons.[64]

The final blow came in 1975 when the Nu Deal consortium put the club's land up for sale two years before the lease expired. Meadowbrook did have two more seasons before the land was finally sold, but on 13 March 1977 twelve members—the same number that started the club—met to count the results of a mail-in vote. Three fourths voted to dissolve the club. Some members drifted back to Sunny Trails, some joined the Hyperions, and others went their separate way.[65]

In June 1972 several members of Meadowbrook broke away to form an independent travel club, the Hyperions. The founders had been members of Meadowbrook since 1968; Ron served as president from 1969 to 1971. In his own club Ron would serve as president for nearly a decade, 1972-75 and 1976-83. As a travel club, Hyperions had its share of members who regarded the quaint rules and regulations of landed clubs as petty annoyances which were beneath them. "We needed a place where there were few rules and a nudist could do whatever he or she wished."[66]

This attitude got the club in trouble on occasion. In 1973 two members visited Sunny Trails, entered without authorization (refusing to reveal how they had learned the gate combination), and engaged in irregular behavior by photographing people with a hidden camera. The host club voted to ban all Hyperions; originally members wanted to ban all travel clubs. The Hyperions discussed the incident at their next meeting, but when the man with the camera explained that he took the pictures because he felt like it, and ignored the camera rules of both clubs because he didn't want to bother reading them, the board let him off with a warning not to get caught again.[67]

After three years of slow but steady growth the first in a series of internal blowups occurred. At a heated meeting in September 1975 the club president was accused of publicly identifying the Hyperions as a swingers club—a charge that he vehemently denied. The club had acquired this image as early as 1974, when a reporter at the Miss Nude Pacific Northwest contest referred to the "mysterious Hyperion group (nudists who swing), but I didn't see any evidence of it. Some pendulosity, but no swinging."[68] Nevertheless, in order to alleviate members' concerns, Ron resigned. Scarcely had his replacement taken office than club members challenged him by club members for a conflict of interest because he and three other Hyperion members had started another travel club, the Totems, which also acquired a reputation for swinging. In February 1976 the board reappointed the first president, and the following month a special session of the board elected a new executive, headed by the founder. By summer the Hyperions appeared to have put this incident behind them, although the publicity director admitted that it was "difficult to promote a good public relationship when we have unrest and strife right here in our own realm."[69]

The Hyperions then polarized over personality and policy disputes involving president Ron and publicity director Korky. Although relatively minor matters were at stake, such as responsibility for guests and for children at club functions, the real issue was personality. Ron, while endorsing individual freedom in a "Liberal Do-your-own-thing Club," preferred to operate according to procedure, while Korky interpreted democracy to mean anarchy.[70] The ensuing commotion split club opinion, resulting in a one-third drop in membership and a clean sweep of the board in 1978. This did not settle the matter, however, and the "Korky issue" came up for discussion repeatedly throughout 1979, with members voting against reinstating him in February, then voting to drop all charges in June and to issue an apology, only to reverse this decision in November by voting to expel him from the club.

But when Ron tried to expel Korky from the WCSA and the ASA the WCSA president questioned his motive: "is self and selfish pride so important to you that you will risk everything you purport to stand for?" As the club secretary tersely remarked, "this past year your board has had more 'set backs' than 'go aheads'."[71]

At the annual membership meeting in November 1980, none of the eleven members who bothered to attend was willing to stand for office. The meeting was postponed until the new year, and once again the founder stepped forward to save the club, "provided that I have complete say in the operation of the Club. . . . The original idea of a co-operative, democratic, altruistic club obviously did not work." He suggested a constitutional amendment to make the Hyperions a proprietary travel club. This was approved unanimously at the February meeting.[72]

Unfortunately, even this drastic step did not save the club. Apathy continued to hold sway over club activities; only one third of the membership attended the club's tenth anniversary party in 1982. Members clearly regarded the Hyperions as a passport to landed clubs, and the president seemed preoccupied with ASA politics. In 1983 the club repeated its 1981 stratagem: Ron stepped aside, and transferred the club to another member, Walt, who valiantly carried on until he too had to confess inability "to guess what you, as members, want." In 1993 a new board reorganized the club as the Vancouver Sunbathing Association, and immediately found itself in trouble with the WCSA, which renamed itself the Western Canadian Association for Nude Recreation in 1994 and insisted on imposing its politically correct new name on all of its affiliated clubs.[73]

CHAPTER FOUR

Raw Hides

The Canadian prairies are anything but flat farmland. The three western provinces—Alberta, Saskatchewan, and Manitoba—are laced with rivers, lakes, and deep forests that allow residents and visitors to get away and enjoy nature. By the 1920s and 1930s many did so in a completely natural way. Even in the far north, in the Yukon (Whitehorse) and the Northwest Territories (Yellowknife, Norman Wells), there have been nudists willing to take advantage of the brief but hot summers to sun and swim—though not enough to form the "Arctic Bares."[1]

Edmonton, surrounded by many secluded lakes, has been home to more nudist clubs over a longer period of time than any other Canadian city. One of the first Albertans who responded to Ray Connett's "Sunny Trails" column reported that "I used to go nude bathing in the lake and often thought how nice it would be to join a club and bathe nude with others." The first organized club appeared in the mid-1920s, but even though the lawyer-founder drafted its rules and regulations, uncertainty among members and lack of sympathy among city authorities led to the rapid demise of this group. A decade later another group took shape and enjoyed several outings until a vice scandal rocked Edmonton in the mid-1930s. Although none of its members was involved, the club chose to fade away. Both groups used Big Island in the North Saskatchewan River for some of their outings.[2]

At the end of the 1930s a group of friends and relatives began sunbathing at a summer cottage owned by a professional couple with nudist experience in Europe and the United States. After awhile the issue of accepting outsiders provoked a split as the members who refused to go public packed up and moved to a new location 100 miles away, leaving the rest to their own devices. And so Edmonton's third nudist group, the AL-ber-TANS, came to an end.[3]

In 1947 Al Travers contacted Ray Connett to inquire about starting a new club in the Edmonton area. Travers met with a former member of the 1930s group who joined the new club, called Edmontans. As Connett referred more prospects, a sizable group took shape. Travers obtained the use of an isolated farm about 80 miles outside Edmonton, but the distance and the difficult access led to a wider search, which produced a "beautiful spot on a huge lake" only 50 miles from town. On Labor Day weekend, 1949, the Edmontans hosted several outside visitors, including the Calgary singles organizer, Alf. Then, in December 1951, Al Travers died, and "two religious daughters burned every scrap of nudist material in the house! . . . Thus a club died with its leader." As the secretary lamented, "we Edmontans owned nothing. The films, books, accounts, etc. were all burned. . . . There was nothing left."[4]

Edmonton still had nudists. In the early 1950s a large singles group with "a good bunch of fellows" was active, using a field a few miles out of town. Its leader had experience dating back to the 1930s. And a few years later a new couple, Charles and Evelyn, contacted Connett about reviving the Edmontans. Another small group existed in Mannville. Then, in January 1956, members of the Edmonton and Mannville groups got together to elect officers and revive the Edmontans. They elected the officers but failed to revive the club.[5]

In 1958 Edmonton nudists got a new chance when another former Edmontanner contacted Connett. The CSA offered Walter their list of past members and current prospects, along with hope for "all the good luck that people need in forming a group in Edmonton." Although Walter was soon transferred to the Northwest Territories on business, he left the club, the Noraltans, in good shape. By the summer of 1959 the Noraltans had forty members and leased land surrounding a 55-acre lake perfectly suited for nude waterskiing (even though the mosquitoes "flew in squadron formation"), along with the more conventional swimming and fishing. The Noraltans continued to use this location for several years, and affiliated with the WCSA/ASA in 1962. Then yet another Edmonton club hijacked them.[6]

In 1963 Dieter Wesemann, a German immigrant, arrived in Edmonton and contacted the Noraltans. Although he associated with them for awhile, his ambition and philosophy led him to set up a rival club which he named Helios Edmonton. During the autumn and winter of 1963-64 a group of interested people met to draw up a constitution. At the same time the club acquired land north of Edmonton. Wesemann encouraged members to contribute time, effort, and money to develop "their" club; later it would become "his" farm.[7]

At first Wesemann organized club activities for Helios Edmonton. Public relations included newspaper advertising and interviews with the newspapers and radio stations and magazines, all of which brought in thirty inquiries per week. Club members enjoyed weekly sauna nights in rented facilities during the winter, to which they added swimming at the YMCA in 1968. In summer they benefitted from an increasing array of facilities at the camp near Westlock, including an artificial pond, above-ground pool, horseshoes, and a children's playground. Many long-lasting friendships, business partnerships, and even marriages formed during these seasons of "wonderful, beautiful summer living" which brought members together. In 1970 the club prepared to host the next WCSA convention.[8]

In 1971 tensions between Wesemann and club members reached the boiling point. Although they all got along reasonably well during the 1960s, Wesemann's autocratic behavior became more and more pronounced. Members who had contributed time, effort, and money to develop the club were eased, squeezed, and pushed out, and Wesemann came to regard the camp as his personal fiefdom. "As long as you said 'yes, master' he was great." He obtained exclusive title to the land, and refused to compensate members who had contributed money and materials for the club. When members started discussing the problems they found themselves banned from camp. Gradually a shadow Helios club took shape and became known as the 1398s after the post office box they rented when Wesemann intercepted all mail sent to the official box 222, even though he was neither president nor secretary.[9]

On 9 November 1971, Helios members held a special meeting to discuss the future of the club. They reaffirmed their commitment to a cooperative structure, and decided that anyone (such as a landowner) with a financial interest in the club could not be an officer but could sit on the board to represent his interests. Wesemann, who attended the meeting, declared that he would ignore the 90 per cent majority vote, so the club voted to suspend him from the board and end his "dictatorial control."[10]

Helios 1398 called the annual meeting for 15 February 1972 to discuss recent developments, elect officers, and plan club activities for the coming year. Chief among their concerns was a new camp, since by now they had all been banned from the old one. An offer of land in nearby Sherwood Park fell through, so the board arranged for members to use the facilities of Glenden Park and Canyon Valley, and to visit Sunny Chinooks in Calgary. At the end of that summer they arranged for winter swims and saunas.[11]

The careful, responsible work of Helios 1398 paid off. Current members retained their affiliation, and past members who had left or formed splinter groups such as Glenden Park returned to the fold. Even erstwhile Wesemann loyalists who had stayed with him in Helios 222 gradually transferred to the 1398 group. Meanwhile, the legal dispute between Wesemann and Helios Edmonton made its way through the courts (as did a bitter divorce and custody battle). Eventually the court ruled against both parties and placed a lien on the former campsite. For his part Wesemann left Edmonton permanently.[12]

Throughout the early 1970s, despite court battles and the loss of their campground, Helios continued to operate as a social club.

Members found that they liked each other, and their troubles with Wesemann "glued them together through friendship." Unlike most other clubs, however, they found that winter was their most active season, with weekly swims, saunas, and fitness activities at area gyms, principally the West Edmonton YMCA. Occasionally, they held inter-club volleyball competitions with Sunny Chinooks members. It was during the summers that the tenuous position of the club took its toll. Although they arranged visits to other local campgrounds (Glenden Park and Canyon Valley) it became increasingly obvious that "without a doubt there is a definite need to have a place that we can call our own."[13]

Finally, in 1978, two member couples found a heavily wooded site 30 miles east of Edmonton near Tofield, and formed a partnership (TaHa Holdings) to buy the land for club use. Later, one couple sold its interest to the other, making the Harrisons exclusive landlords. In 1990 they sold the land to another couple who carried on for a few years before moving to British Columbia. Meanwhile another couple dropped out in an abortive effort to start the Northern Sands club. In 1994 Helios Edmonton became a cooperative club with 22 acres of wooded land, a heated in-ground pool, sauna, hot tub, and clubhouse, all to accommodate 125 members, who celebrated their thirtieth anniversary in 1995.[14]

Some of the Helios members who grew weary of Wesemann's autocratic behavior broke away in early 1969 and formed the Glenden Park Nudist Society. In May they rented land west of Edmonton, near Jackfish Lake, from a sympathetic farmer, and the fifty members enjoyed volleyball, horseshoes, archery, and swimming in a 15-acre lake. Members also visited other clubs. In winter Glenden Park held meetings and parties in members' homes, and sponsored biweekly swims at the Victoria Composite High School, which proved amenable after other institutions had difficulty conceptualizing nude swimming.[15]

Back at camp, although club relations with the farmer landlord remained good, this was not the case with his sons, and members found themselves subject to harassment from voyeurs and vandals. 1972 was the last season at camp. By now Helios was stable, if still landless, and most Glenden Park members returned to the fold along with other Wesemann waifs. They all found a summer haven at Canyon Valley. Still others formed the short-lived Hill and Dale travel club.[16]

Several other smaller clubs have operated in Edmonton over the years. In 1968 a couple living near Wetaskiwin proposed to start a club to serve the area south of Edmonton, but this group remained a small circle of friends without WCSA affiliation. In the mid-1970s a former Amway entrepreneur, Dennis Egger, launched three clubs to cater to a variety of life-styles. The Edmonton Suntanners Lodge sponsored a Miss Nude Edmonton contest to showcase the exotic dancers of the Chez Pierre nightclub. The Edmonton Running Bares organized indoor swims for its predominantly male membership at the Victoria Composite High School. Egger also claimed responsibility for the Edmonton Gymnosophical Society, but his own legal problems took him away from organizational work, and all three clubs folded.[17]

In 1977 the Altans group was started by veteran nudists who were former operators of the Conjuring Park free beach camp at Wizard Lake. They organized indoor activities at the West Edmonton Y, including swimming and inter-club volleyball competition. But once the reformed Helios club obtained land in 1978 the Altans disbanded.[18]

In 1984 the Edmonton Nudist Society formed as a non-landed club to provide nudist recreation to people "whose lifestyles, jobs, situations, etc., don't permit them to make the more extensive commitment necessary to make joining a landed club worthwhile." They organized indoor swimming and saunas at the Bonnie Doon pool and at the Grand Trunk pool, which had a unique kiddie pool and a jacuzzi. TENS remained active after its founder transferred to Kamloops, until lack of interest compelled the board to dissolve the club at the end of 1993.[19]

In 1947 a "lone nudist" from Calgary contacted Ray Connett in

Sunbathing for Health magazine. A few other nudists gradually identified themselves, and by 1950 two small groups formed: one for single men, another for couples. Both took advantage of the nearby Bow River valley for sunbathing. (Calgary teens had their own spot south of the MacDonald Bridge.) In 1951 Alf, the singles leader, agreed to work with Bob, the couples leader, and the following year the two groups cooperated on several outings to an isolated spot off the Banff highway. In April 1952 the couples group, hitherto known as the Chinook Sunshine Club, absorbed many of the singles and restyled itself Sunny Chinooks.[20]

During the 1950s Sunny Chinooks was unusually peripatetic. For awhile they continued to use the farm near the Banff Highway, six miles west of Calgary. In 1955 they leased land along the MacLeod Trail west of Midnapore, 25 miles south of Calgary. Early in 1956 they found a spot closer to the city, but urban sprawl necessitated a constant lookout, so they packed up again and moved to the southwest foothills near Priddis, where they found a spot that they christened "the Sahara Desert" because it was bone dry (except when it rained). In 1957 they moved one mile west to a more attractive but still dry location.[21]

Just when things looked promising, "internal trouble took a hand and blew everything up." Members clashed with the leader, who "had a few strange ideas." He was subsequently expelled from the club and the CSA for "moral and camera reasons." In 1958 only two members remained involved, and their only accomplishment was to rename the club San Helios "in hopes that recent trouble would be forgotten and a fresh start made, but it was a lost cause and the entire organization simply folded up." In June 1959 Ray Connett, visiting Calgary from Vancouver, mediated between the parties and obtained the club's postal box and key from the former leader who disappeared. He resurfaced in 1962 under a new name and tried, unsuccessfully, to rejoin his old club.[22]

When Rod Flack returned to Calgary in 1959 after a lengthy absence, he found the club in disarray. A handful of San Helios members met early in the year to rebuild their club. In April one of them arranged to lease land in Priddis. During his June visit Connett offered advice on club reorganization, and appeared on a Calgary radio station. In July the club voted to change its name back to Sunny Chinooks Association and to adopt the white cowboy hat as its official uniform. Things were looking up again, and members now aspired to become "one of the leading clubs of the west."[23]

Then disaster struck in the form of a sudden cloudburst. Ray Connett had described the road into camp as "a sad series of mudholes," and the club pool as a "bulldozed mudhole," but on 2 August 1959 the whole camp became a mudhole.[24] Throughout the autumn of 1959 the club executive searched for a new campsite. In February 1960 the Land Committee recommended an 89-acre site just west of High River, south of Calgary. It was isolated, well-secluded, and had a serviceable pond for swimming. In spring the club bought the property for $8,000 and prepared to enjoy the first of many summers. Financing the purchase proved difficult for a relatively small club (a mid-summer meeting was attended by "10 adult members, 4 children and 5 dogs"), and in 1961 president Ralph proposed that he or a group of members buy the property and lease it to the club, or that members approve a substantial increase in dues to cover the mortgage payments. "Without a firmer long range policy to which we must adhere, failure must stare us in the face."[25]

The club regrouped long enough to host the 1962 WCSA convention, held for the first time east of the Rockies and timed to coincide with the Calgary Stampede. Members tried to be optimistic, despite their recent experiences.

> There is a club in Calgary
> We'd like you all to come and see
> Sunny Chinooks is our name
> Hospitality is our fame
> Come to the gate with the great big sign
> Highwood Acres on a pine
> People come for miles around

Just to see our beautiful ground
There are nudists in this camp
Most of them were pretty damp
I wish to hell the sun would shine
But it keeps raining all the time
We are stuck up on the hill
Next convention we'll be there still.[26]

By the end of the summer the worsening financial situation led two officers to resign. Members then approved the formation of a syndicate of several members who would buy Highwood Acres and lease it to the Sunny Chinooks Association. Eventually Sunny Chinooks was reorganized so that only the four landowners—Bob, David, Don, and Rod—were "full" members; all others became "associate" members, with no voice in the financial affairs of Highwood Enterprises.[27]

Once again a severe rainstorm flooded the property, breaking the river dike and washing out roads and bridges. Repairs were made, but the club "resolved that the present land be sold and new land acquired." In May 1964 the Sunny Chinooks Association authorized its syndicate, Highwood Enterprises, to negotiate a lease with another company, Leah Properties, on land purchased by Leah Properties outside Cochrane, west of Calgary. The Leah Properties partnership bought 160 acres and sold 120 acres to pay for the remaining 40 acres. In later years the other two partners sold their shares to Rod Flack, who in turn sold about half of that to a neighbor (and club member) in the 1970s. In the meantime Highwood Enterprises acted as trustee for the club. It collected club revenues, paid the lease, and administered capital developments. Among other things, it was obligated to construct a pool on the new land.[28]

Once Sunny Chinooks secured a stable campground it was able to plan for the future. Although it was still a relatively small club (thirty-five adults in 1964), members worked diligently to improve the campground, while enjoying indoor swimming, steam baths, and volleyball at rented facilities in Calgary during the winter. Development at Triple Diamond Ranch (their new campsite) proceeded steadily: above-ground pool (1967), volley-ball court (1969), clubhouse (1970), sauna (1973), in-ground pool (1974), horseshoes, badminton court, children's playground, and whirlpool (1978), relax center with sauna, hot tub, and showers (1982). These improvements, together with regular advertising and feature articles in the *Calgary Herald* (notably for the club's thirtieth anniversary in 1982) helped boost membership from 35 in 1964 to 50 ten years later, to 200 by 1980, and to more than 300 by 1985.[29]

Throughout the 1970s the principal subject of club "politicking and bickering" was the relationship between Leah Properties and the Sunny Chinooks Association. In September 1971, the annual general meeting discussed these issues. Rod Flack declared that "the property would be available for sunbathing purposes for all time" and offered a five year renewable lease. He also affirmed his expectation that the club would remain affiliated with the WCSA/ASA, but members disagreed on this point and voted to give one year's notice of withdrawal. When the time came for the final vote, in November 1972, Flack informed the club that Triple Diamond Ranch would be available only to members of ASA-affil-iated clubs, and Sunny Chinooks was forced to rescind its motion to withdraw.[30]

Perhaps because of Flack's power of ultimatum, members' unrest continued during the 1970s. In 1973 Flack complained that "over the years when members have been asked to contribute a lit-tle bit of muscular effort and yes possibly financial effort, we have heard the stories come back from some club members that 'why should they contribute, they're not even sure they'll be on the land next year.' Some people have used that excuse for years, and quite frankly it's worn itself out." And in 1978 he wrote, "the property known as Triple Diamond Ranch will always be a nudist park. The ground will be my resting place, the trees will be my headstone, and my interest will remain with my remains." Flack made a compelling argument, since his membership went back further than anyone else's and he had saved the club on more than one occasion. Nevertheless, members remained unconvinced. So long as no legal arrangement governed the relationship between tenant and landlord, and so long as the landlord continued to express concern over the rate of return on investment compared with conventional campgrounds, uncertainty prevailed.[31]

One year later Sunny Chinooks finally negotiated a contract with Leah Properties governing future developments. In 1981 the club voted to turn over its assets to Leah Properties and convert Triple Diamond Ranch into an owner-operated resort effective 1 April 1983. (Leah Properties would then become Triple Diamond Ranch Ltd.) SCA remained in place to coordinate social activities and to comply with provincial regulations. This settlement brought a temporary end to internal squabbling as club members celebrated two milestones: the thirtieth anniversary of the Sunny Chinooks Club in 1982 and the twentieth anniversary of Triple Diamond Ranch in 1984.[32]

The 1981 accord barely survived the decade. Financial concerns remained a problem despite—or perhaps because of—the owner's pledge that rates "will remain stable for a number of years." Hints about "going textile" became more frequent, and members felt that they were no longer wanted at their own club. Misunderstandings persisted, as Flack assumed that all of the club's assets and monies were his to use for the development of his Triple Diamond Ranch, while disparaging those contributions as inadequate. By the late 1980s both sides agreed that "the outlook at that time was bleak and the club was generally dispirited. The desperate situation required desperate action to save the club." But the "vicious rumors, half truths, and lies" continued to poison relations. "It is unfortunate that the detrimental covert actions of a few have been the ruination of one of the best Western Canadian nudist clubs, but that is exactly what transpired."[33]

Another factor in the "ruination" of Sunny Chinooks was the changing attitude of Karen Flack towards nudism. Although she joined Sunny Chinooks "because I liked the nude stuff," by the end of the 1980s she had disassociated herself from nudism. And so, in the summer of 1990, after members agreed to transfer funds to finance a new swimming pool, Rod Flack announced that Triple Diamond Ranch would convert to a conventional RV park for 1991. A thirty year association between landlord and tenant came to a regrettable end.[34]

The newly evicted club members wasted little time in regrouping. They continued their tradition of indoor winter swims. More decisively, the club set up a Land and Development trust which quickly accumulated a $15,000 reserve, and appointed a land committee to search for a new campsite. In 1992 Sunny Chinooks acquired $18^1/_2$ acres of wooded land on the James River near Sundre, 130 kilometers northwest of Calgary. It was about as much land as they had at Triple Diamond Ranch, in about the same area. A dozen members pledged to contribute several thousand dollars apiece to finance purchase of the land, and in 1995 the club acquired full ownership of the property and became a cooperative club owned by the membership. Many who left in 1990 have now returned. Considering everything the club has endured, Sunny Chinooks certainly qualifies as the phoenix of Canadian nudist clubs.[35]

When Sunny Chinooks decided to leave Highwood Acres back in 1964 and search for new land, some of the members, led by one of the Highwood Enterprises partners, decided that the time was right to break off and form a separate club, Golden Sun Ranch. This first attempt proved abortive, possibly because Sunny Chinooks found new land so quickly, but some members tried again in 1967 and managed to hold together until the end of the decade, when a change in policy at Sunny Chinooks persuaded most of them to return to the fold.[36]

A few years later the temporary absence of Rod Flack for personal reasons allowed scope to other board members, some of whom held views which differed from those of the majority of members, who complained that the new secretary was able to "flood the club grounds with single males" and to "brainwash the members (especially new ones) to her way of thinking." Growing animosity towards her more "open" nudism led her and her husband to revive Golden Sun Ranch (GSR) as a travel club based at their suburban home. They provided GSR members with a swimming pool, sunning lawn, and sauna, and joined with Sunny Chinooks in sponsoring indoor winter swims. During the summer members visited Sunny Chinooks, Helios, and Canyon Valley. Membership topped sixty by 1974, but with the transfer of Canyon Valley to new owners and the death of Laura Baecker in 1978, Golden Sun lapsed into limbo once again.[37]

The group revived in 1980 on the initiative of former members. They sponsored indoor winter swims and summer visits to other clubs while looking for land of their own. But conflicts of interest among board members thwarted this incarnation also. Then in 1982 another member of Golden Sun who lived in Lethbridge proposed a club there to serve southern Alberta. The Wheatland Sun Club attracted local members of Sunny Chinooks as well as newcomers. It offers indoor swimming in the winter and arranged group visits to Sunny Chinooks until that club reorganized in 1990.[38]

In November 1948 a promising contact from Regina wrote to Ray Connett to arrange a meeting with the local CSA group leader, Bob. Andy owned 1400 acres on Last Mountain Lake, including a mile of shoreline and nicely wooded land.

> All summer when I had the chance I would go down
> to the Lake and discard me clothing, take a dip in Lake
> and lie down or walk among the trees. I have never
> felt better in my life than I have felt this last summer.[39]

Andy offered this land for the use of the Regina group without obligation. Ray put the two men in touch, and they started to cooperate, although Bob had more restrictive ideas regarding single members than Andy would have liked. Both were determined that "there will be no scandal" among the "very narrow-minded" people in the area. Unfortunately, nothing came of this initiative, and Regina would not see another group until the 4-S Club in the early 1960s, and that too would be shortlived.[40]

Further north, an active group of about twenty met in members' homes in Saskatoon during the late 1940s and used one member's farm on a river south of town during the summers. But when he moved to Ontario in 1952 the club dissolved. Other nudists tried to maintain cohesion by correspondence until a new club could be formed.[41]

In 1958 a young, single Saskatoon architect formed the Havatan Park club. The group started small and remained small because the owner insisted on secrecy to protect his professional identity. "Jim," the club president, owned 160 acres of bush along a winding river, "one of the finest nudist properties we have yet visited." The camp provided limited swimming in the river, badminton, and archery. After a decade of slow growth bordering on stagnation, and after two visits by Ray Connett, who appeared on local radio, the club did start to organize indoor winter activities, including monthly swim nights and volleyball.[42]

Although Havatan Park affiliated with the WCSA/ASA in 1970, it remained suspicious of outside contact, and very quickly found cause for grievance when some members left to start the new Prairie Suntan Society, and one of those members became Provincial Director for the WCSA. In 1975 the club distanced itself from the WCSA, blaming procedural wrangles and "unwarranted remarks by the Provincial Director," and the next year members voted to quit the WCSA/ASA "as no benefit is derived from the WCSA."[43]

Jim's personality affected not only the club's external relations with the WCSA, but internal relations as well. Since Havatan Park was one of the few nudist clubs owned and operated by a single man, some of the married men felt uneasy about bringing their wives to camp or leaving them there alone. Jim also became increasingly assertive as landowner, vetoing actions of the club board affecting his land. Membership defections to Prairie Suns and later to Green Haven further weakened the club, and in the 1980s Jim dissolved the club and retired to live on his land.[44]

In 1972 "a few couples here in Saskatoon have decided to form a new sunbathing club." The Prairie Suntan Society started with the intention of becoming a landed club, and rented land for 1973. But the founder did not promote the club well enough to support a landed camp, and in 1978 it settled into the travel club routine as the Prairie Suns, visiting the new Green Haven club in Regina (which was also formed by disgruntled Havatans) and spending winter vacations in "sunnier climes."[45]

Events in Saskatoon produced a new Regina club, Green Haven. In the early 1970s the Prairie Suns rented property near Saskatoon. When the lease expired, some of the Regina-based members reconsidered the four-hour round-trip drive every week-end. Werner and Karin decided to shop around, and in 1973 they leased some land in the Qu'appelle Valley from relatives. Green Haven Sun Club was born, and affiliated with the WCSA. In 1977 the owners of the land sold out, and for a year Green Haven became a travel club just like Prairie Suns. But Werner was busy again, and in 1978 he purchased land east of Regina and made 25 acres available to the club.[46]

Green Haven grew through publicity, organization, and dedi-cation. The club used newspaper ads and occasional household flier drops to attract inquiries. They also invite media coverage, including TV, especially when they host regional conventions. In 1980 CKVT-TV filmed a documentary on nudism and broadcast it twice because of popular demand. Club members also speak at the university and the public library, where they have donated books and videos on nudism. Club activities include winter swims, bowling, and social gatherings in members' homes. At camp they use the newly expanded Nudaplex clubhouse, above-ground swimming pool, sauna, volleyball and badminton courts, and a children's playground with swings, bars, playhouse, and sandbox. If starting a nudist club is like betting on the lottery, Green Haven has hit the jackpot in more ways than one. The unique and friendly ambience of the club is well appreciated by visitors, particularly at WCSA conventions.[47]

Manitoba naturists are blessed with two huge inland lakes

with fine sandy beaches, myriad smaller lakes, rivers, woods, and what passes for mountains east of the Rockies. In the 1930s individuals and couples went out to Lake Winnipeg for sun and health, canoed down the Assiniboine and Red rivers, or travelled further north to Riding Mountain National Park. "We swam around listlessly and never have I enjoyed water and freedom so much." But outside of the metropolis attempts to organize clubs failed—perhaps because there was no need for a "club" when Nature was all around.[48]

In 1948 John and Anne gathered together a local group of enthusiasts which became the Manitoba Outdoor Club (MOC) in 1949. Winter became the most active season for the club because of failure to find a campsite. When the club first considered land they let their imagination run wild: "We hope to buy a full section of land—640 acres—and develop it as a site for a permanent all-weather club house, a recreational area, a playground for our kiddies, a parking space for trailers, and to build a few cabins for out-of-town guests." But a club with only a dozen members could hardly afford to buy and develop a square mile of land, so they scaled down their field of dreams to a mere quarter section—but a quarter section with a clear, deep, wide river flowing right through it that would be the focal point of a residential complex and recreation center. The whole operation would be financed by the sale of shares entitling members to a long-term lease on their own cabin sites. But unfortunately this vision also fell through.[49]

Land remained a problem until 1960 when a club member made his summer cottage site on Lake Winnipeg near Beaconia available for club use. Until then, the club met biweekly for combined business and social meetings featuring indoor miniature golf, balloon volleyball, carpet croquet, cards, bingo, and sing-alongs, all under the beneficial glare of sunlamps to make indoor nudism worthwhile.[50]

During the 1950s the Manitoba Outdoor Club lived up to its name by spending summer weekends travelling for outings to secluded beaches on Lake Winnipeg and Lake Manitoba and to isolated spots such as the Brokenhead and Fisher rivers. Starting with twenty prospects in 1949, the club declined steadily until 1956, when only three paid memberships graced the club register. As late as 1959 MOC continued to lament that "our difficulty is finding a suitable spot for our outdoor activities." But the very next year a recent member, Art, bought ten acres on the east shore of Lake Winnipeg near Beaconia which he made available as the club campsite.[51]

Tan Acres was "a beautiful spot" with volleyball and badminton courts, horseshoes, and swings for the children. Having a fixed address at long last—even if the club itself did not own or control the land—helped foster growth, and membership rose to a peak of forty-three adults and sundry children. In 1972 the club revived its earlier practice of indoor winter meetings by renting swimming pools from the YMCA, with MOC providing its own lifeguard. The club also started to advertise systematically, even presenting a radio phone-in show in 1971 that generated its very own crank caller who asked irately if somewhat illogically, "Are those people sitting there naked?" MOC also used feature articles and regular newspaper ads, which brought in more than one hundred inquiries, and sponsored the screening of an ASA promotional video on a local cable station.[52]

When Art gave the club use of his campground, matters began to look up again, and the secretary wrote to the CSA regarding affiliation. But this time the CSA itself was splitting apart into separate organizations, so once again "nothing has been decided yet." Not until 1966 would MOC join the WCSA.[53]

The 1970s marked the beginning of the end for the club. For years many members had been growing dissatisfied with Tan Acres because of the lack of facilities, especially for children; the increasing summer population in the area, which compelled them to flee the beach at regular intervals; the gender imbalance due to "a disproportionate number of male singles"; and the lack of club control over "its" land. In 1968 a new member, Leon, represented MOC at the WCSA convention in British Columbia. At the host

Meadowbrook club he saw what a "real" nudist club looked like, with its full array of recreational facilities and activities. When he returned to MOC his request for similar facilities at Tan Acres was rejected by the owner. In 1969 Leon and several other members, including John and Anne, the founders of MOC, left Tan Acres to start a new club with "facilities, atmosphere, and suitable grounds conducive to family nudism."[54]

Crocus Grove started as a cooperative club, but some of the original participants grew alarmed at the scope of the work that lay ahead of them and quit, so in 1973 Crocus Grove was restructured as a proprietary club with Leon as sole owner.

Noting that cooperative clubs tended to languish while proprietary clubs forged ahead, and believing that "a benevolent dictatorship is not always a bad thing," Leon and Evelyn took over all operations in 1973 and quickly inaugurated major improvements, including an in-ground swimming pool, sauna, and hot showers. Membership continued to grow through active publicity in the media and at the university. The club televised the ASA video "The Take-Off" on cable, and has received live TV coverage whenever it hosts WCSA conventions.[55]

Crocus Grove Sun Club is situated on 60 sandy acres of heavily wooded land about 40 miles north of Winnipeg and is accessible by expressway and paved secondary roads (a novelty for a nudist camp). An impressive two-story clubhouse with hot tub and sauna serves as the centerpiece. An extensive children's playground features swings, teeter totters, sandbox, and other playground equipment which are put to special use during the occasional Olympic Days competitions for children and adults.[56]

Swimming remains a popular winter activity, and the club continues renting a pool at the Y where about half of the members attend regularly—except on the night the Y double-booked them with a church group. (Each group eschewed converting the other and the nudists retired to a member's home for hot tubbing.) Crocus Grove has also arranged a charter cruise to small islands in

Lake Winnipeg near Gimli in the spirit of the original MOC. In 1994 it celebrated its twenty-fifth anniversary with guests from across Western Canada and neighboring states. Previously, in a fitting tribute to the place Crocus Grove holds in Western Canada, the club hosted the silver anniversary of the WCSA in 1985.[57]

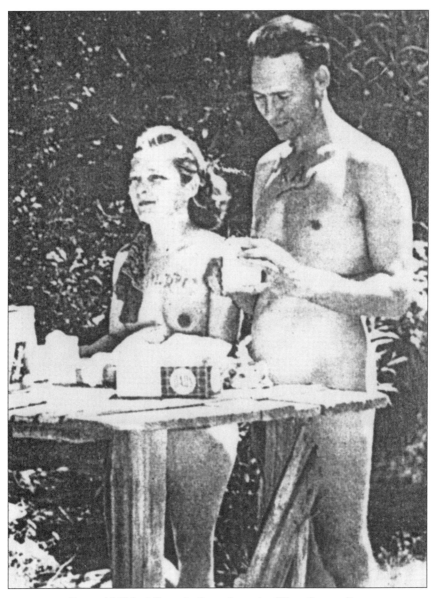

Ray and Mildred Connett, the godparents of Canadian nudism.

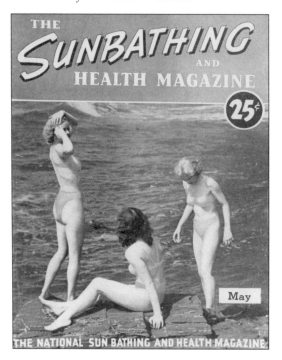

Sunbathing and Health, *Canada's public nudist magazine. The photo shows the cover of the first issue, May 1939.*

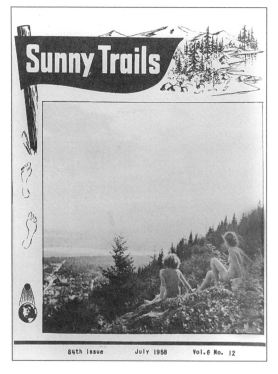

Sunny Trails, *Connett's magazine, later* Canadian Sun Air. *The cover shows the view from the Van Tan Club.*

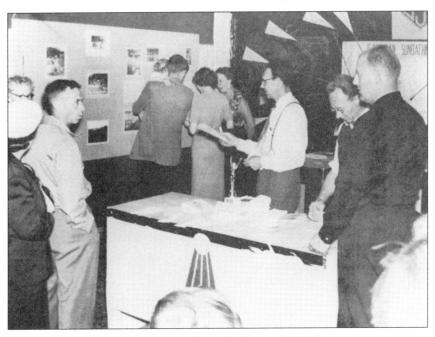

The CSA booth at the Pacific National Exhibition.

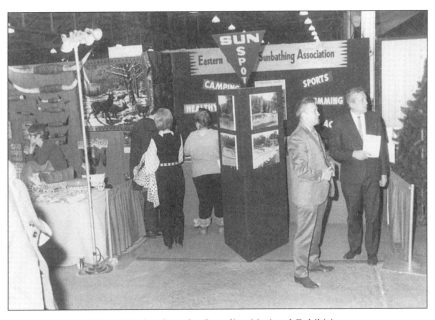

The ECSA booth at the Canadian National Exhibition.

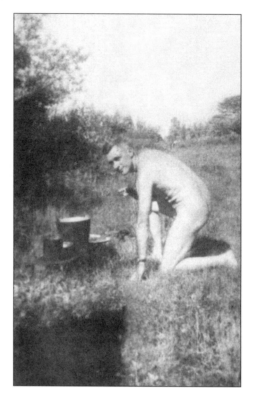

Marcus Meed, founder of the Maritans and CSA president.

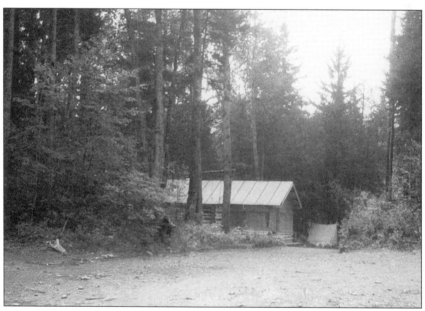

The Maritans campsite outside Bristol, NB.

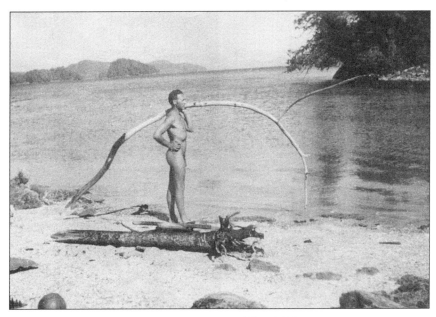

Ray Connett at Port Alberni, BC.

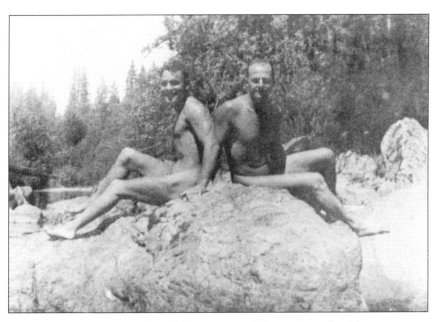

Vancouver Island Health & Hygiene Club. Mex is on the right.

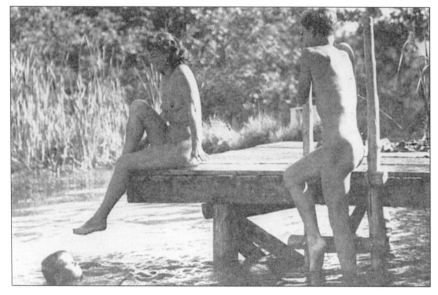

On the dock at Sol Sante.

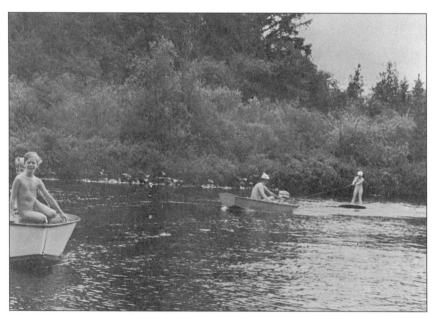

Waterskiing at Sol Sante.

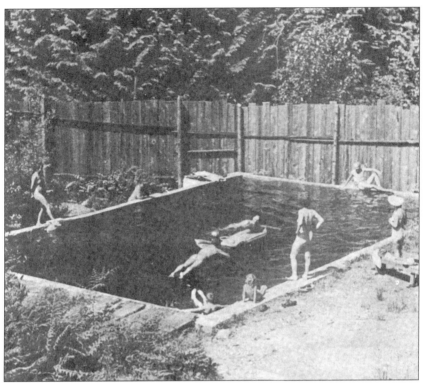

The swimming pool at the Van Tan Club.

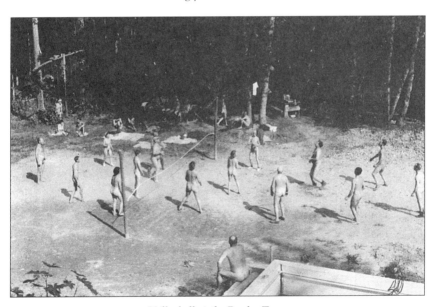

Volleyball at the Border Tans.

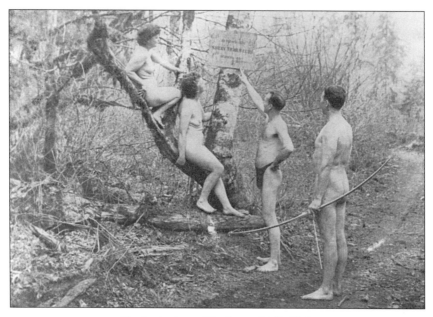

The beginnings of the Sunny Trails Club.

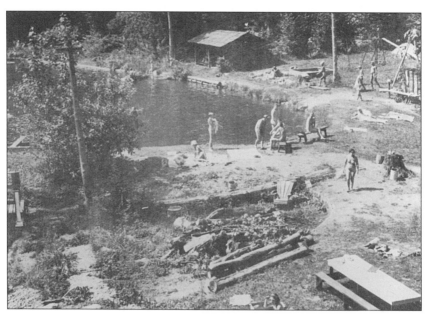

The "construction camp atmosphere" at Sunny Trails.

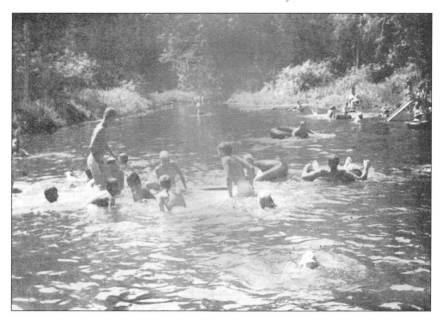

Swimming in Walker Lake at Sunny Trails.

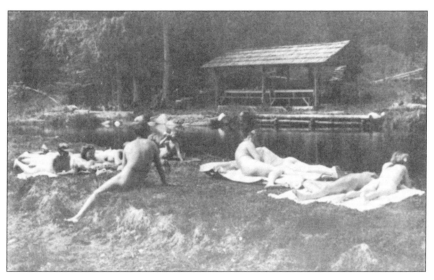

Rest & Relaxation at Sunny Trails.

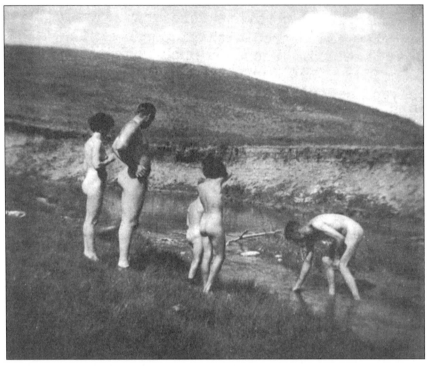

An early Sunny Chinooks outing in the Bow River valley.

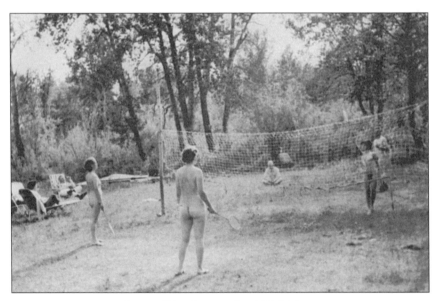

Sunny Chinooks campsite at High River.

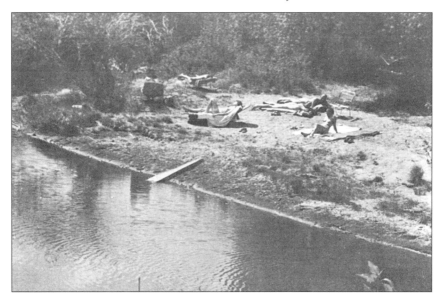

The Havatans campsite near Saskatoon.

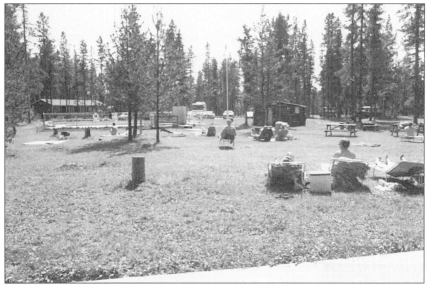

Sunny Chinooks at Triple Diamond Ranch near Cochrane, AB.

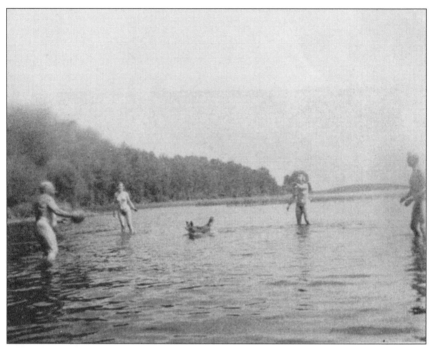

The Edmontans camp on a lake near Edmonton.

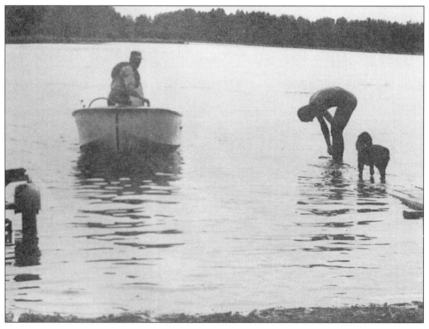

The Noraltans camp on a lake near Edmonton.

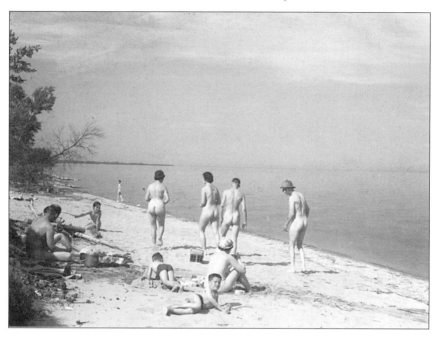

The Manitoba Outdoor Club on the beach along Lake Winnipeg.

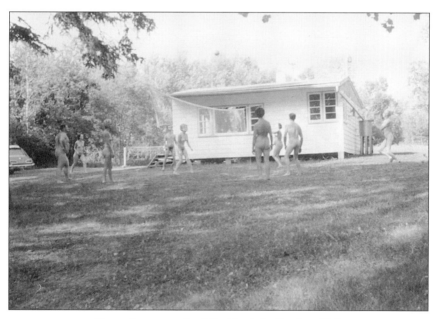

The modern campsite of the Manitoba Outdoor Club.

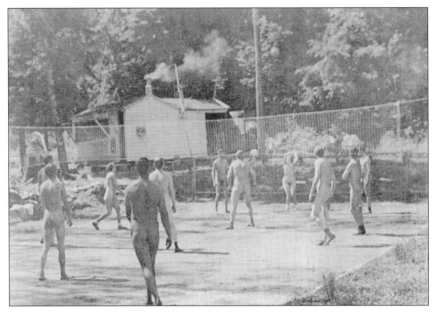

CSA 1958 convention volleyball at Sunny Trails.

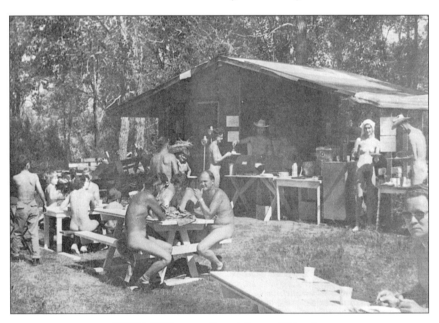

WCSA 1962 convention at Sunny Chinooks.

CHAPTER FIVE

Dawn in the East

Ontario is often called vacation country, and many of its popular resort areas attract naturists. Whether sailing in Georgian Bay, hiking on the Bruce Trail, or camping in Algonquin Park, Ontarians have long found opportunity to "enjoy many happy hours swimming nude."

> I enjoy the out-of-doors very much. The summer never seems complete until I have spent at least a weekend in Northern Ontario's lake district, where one can feel completely free of city convention and prying eyes. My best vacations have been spent on canoe trips in the Lake Temagami district. A rugged "nature" trip seems to be the most invigorating and recreative thing one can do.[1]

Not all northern nudism is of the wilderness type, however. Minaki Lodge had its own informal nudist club circa 1940 with year-round skinny dipping, thanks to a secret pipeline from the Lodge boilers to a nearby secluded lake.

> While it never grew to a vast size, it included several of the permanent members of the Lodge's staff, various Lodge employees who spent singles summers there (it is a popular place of employment for Varsity students during their holidays), and, occasionally, guests of the Lodge.[2]

The Sun-Air-Freedom-Lovers (SAFL), Ontario's first official club, started during the war, when a "very broad-minded couple" from Owen Sound placed an ad in *Sunbathing for Health* asking "Ontario naturists over thirty, interested in arranging lakeside holiday during spring or summer months," to contact them. By the early 1940s there were many Canadians who read nudist magazines, and enough of them contacted Walter to justify the experiment of renting a summer camp in central Ontario. In 1943, 1946, and 1947 they rented Bald's Island off the southern tip of Robert's Island in Georgian Bay, out of Honey Harbour. In 1944 and 1945 they picked "an island in a beautiful lake." Each season seemed better than the one before.[3]

In 1945 the camp at Rice Lake, near Peterborough, was "on an island which looked like a jewel on the water with miles of sparkling lake surrounding it." Facilities included a cottage which served as the clubhouse, canoes, sail boats and motor boats, volleyball, badminton, ping pong, swimming, and fishing. This year the group officially organized on a club basis. Walter, the founder, became the first president. Sun Air had its own newsletter, the *Link*, which kept members in contact during the long months between camps.[4]

In 1946 SAFL returned to Georgian Bay. A pleasant mix of "good company and games and K.P. and everything, not forgetting the Polkas," made the 1946 season "the best yet." For months afterwards members wrote in to recall "the best holiday we ever had," how they enjoyed "the grandest relaxation," how they "hated to leave." One member even wrote a poem in tribute while on board the *City of Midland* heading home.

> Once again to thee, Belle Isle
> I give a farewell wave
> But with a very grateful smile
> Of mem'ries g'lore to rave.[5]

Although the summers at camp provided an enjoyable experience, members were growing weary of not having their own permanent camp, a place where they would be safe from intrusions—such as "the party of fisherfolk that came into our dock to request drinking water" and caused a "frantic scramble for clothes"—and free from prying eyes, such as the man armed with "an excellent pair of binoculars" who complained to police that "we were swimming and diving from our dock completely nude."[6]

For these reasons SAFL decided in late 1946 to search for property of their own. But when it became clear that they would not find a camp in time for the 1947 season, members agreed to return to "our beloved 'Belle Isle'," which provided occasion for one more memorable moment when Hazel McKague borrowed a sailboat to go for groceries. While docking she slipped and fell in the water, and the boat drifted away. Ever resourceful, she swam after it, grabbed the rope in her teeth, and swam back to shore with boat in tow.[7]

In summer 1948 SAFL acquired its own campground, thanks to Bob Babcock, a new member from North Bay. Bob had been trying to stir up interest in nudism in his home town on the pages of *Sunbathing for Health*, particularly among the seventy local people who bought the magazine each month in North Bay; he believed that "there must be some who are sincerely interested in naturism." When Bob accepted the new position of the club secretary, he told members that "you expect your secretary to provide a camp for you," and that he did when he found "a veritable Naturist dreamland"—100 acres of birch trees on a "small but beautiful lake," just outside North Bay. Another member purchased an additional 300 acres, and, together with surrounding crown land, the Sun Air club had 1,200 acres of virtually unlimited privacy (except for the time when some escaped convicts hid out in the bush. But they had precedent on their side since the land had been used as a POW camp during the war.)[8]

The Sun-Air camp centered on Otter Lake, which offered swimming, boating, sailing, and water skiing on two square miles of clear blue water—"not exactly a puddle." The main campsite was set in one of the many coves along the lakeshore, and that is where the clubhouse and games courts for volleyball, badminton, and shuffleboard would be built. The bunkhouse perched on top of a ridge overlooking the lake. The setting and the facilities appealed to all who appreciated a true outdoors camp: "the grounds and lake are just as Mother Nature planned them."[9]

The move to North Bay changed the ambience of the Sun Air club irretrievably. When summer camp had to be specially arranged each year at a rented island location, the ensuing sense of adventure generated group enthusiasm. Everyone appreciated camp as a special privilege which they could not otherwise experience without travelling to the United States (which some did anyhow, especially to Florida in the winter). But when the club accepted the North Bay location as its permanent home, far removed from the "Muskoka mystique" of Georgian Bay and the Kawarthas, camp lost some of its magic. Now the disadvantages of a long trek to the far north weighed against the admitted benefits of a beautiful but isolated home base. Gradually, imperceptibly at first, the character of the club shifted from a seasonal vacation center attracting nudists from all of eastern Canada (the most distant active member lived in Cape Breton) to an established but local club serving North Bay. And there simply were not enough avowed nudists in North Bay to support a permanent landed club.[10]

The Sun-Air club set out to build positive relations with the local community. In the summer of 1949 members invited neighboring families for a day of summertime activity, including swimming, games, dancing, and a sing-along around the campfire, with hot dogs and roasted marshmallows. That same summer the *North Bay Daily Nugget* sent a team to prepare a feature article about the camp. Both the reporter and the photographer were "struck with the beauty of the lake" and wasted no time enjoying "their first nude swim since they were kids." They respected the anonymity of members and took only pictures approved by club representatives. "The next day the story appeared, and it was wonderful. It was a story that money could not buy. . . ."[11]

In the spring of 1950 SAFL came up with a new name. Because of the publicity given to the Doukhobor sect the Sons of Freedom, and because Cold War Canada experienced its own McCarthyism, the term "Freedom Lovers" became suspect, and members concluded that a change was desirable. They also proposed that the CSA formally ban communists, but the national sunbathing organization was not sufficiently alarmed by that kind of red menace and rejected the motion. None the less, in 1950 the "Sun-Air-Freedom-Lovers" became "Norhaven" because "we do have a real naturist haven and it is located in the north of Ontario."[12]

SAFL/Norhaven was financed by shares that members could buy in $100 units. But shareholding was not compulsory, and the majority opted for associate membership, with annual dues and daily or weekly ground (admission) fees. This helped to meet routine operating expenses but did nothing to pay off the mortgage or to finance improvements, such as the clubhouse, dormitory, and rental cabins. To encourage development, the club decided in 1949 to allow members to lease individual campsites where they could build their own cabin or cottage. Eventually the club hoped to see "our lake bordered by a fair-sized naturist community."[13]

The secretary became the focal point of all debate within the club. Bob rubbed people the wrong way from day 1. No sooner had he joined the Sun-Air club and accepted office than he wrote: "in the short time that I have been Sect. Treas., I have received much censure and little support." Although in 1948 members expressed "our sincere appreciation to Bob and Florence for the splendid work they have done during the past year," and even though they reelected Bob as secretary, he soon quarrelled with the acting president (for not acting) and resigned, "to maintain conflict free relations within the club." In 1949 he declined to stand for election in the club, and nearly quit the CSA.[14]

Bob felt that the things that he did as secretary—corresponding with applicants, writing articles for magazines, arranging media publicity—"do not show and that is the reason I have not got credit for them, the things that show are the manual jobs that have improved the camp grounds." In 1951, when he declined to stand as secretary, he reminded his critics that, "despite what you seem to think of me, despite how little some credit me with for anything, you would not have one of the world's finest naturist camps today if I had done other than I have." Feeling no strong support from either members or fellow officers, Bob told Connett that he would withdraw from the club. "I'm not like you Ray, I can't keep turning the other cheek."[15]

By 1952 the rift between the secretary and the rest of the club, led by Bill Irvine, the property manager, became final. Feeling that the manager and his wife "seem to just have taken over," Bob assumed the worst: "I cannot help but see the end of Norhaven in sight." In fact, at the 1954 annual meeting the president and vice president received permission from the shareholding members to buy the shares and assume private ownership and full responsibility for the club. The following year Bob retreated to a cabin on his private island at the far end of the lake and withdrew from club life officially. But it was an open lake, and over the years many members drove or sailed down to Bob's camp, which became an alternative club within the club.[16]

In 1959 the president, Bill, bought out his partner, Hugh, who moved down to Bob's corner of the lake and built his own camp on Bob's launching ramp. This did not improve club finances either, and by 1962 the Irvines started thinking of selling out completely. The rugged outdoor life did not appeal to everyone, and over the years many visitors became disenchanted with the cold air, cold water, hungry blackflies, and the perpetually rustic accommodations. Facilities had not improved yet fees kept rising. Members had more choice as clubs developed in Toronto and Niagara. In 1963 Norhaven closed its gates, twenty years after the first SAFL members gathered to offer Ontario nudists "sunshine, air, and freedom." Today all that remains is Bob's cabin, the cement shuffleboard court, and one beautiful lake.[17]

The spirit of Norhaven lived on briefly in three other northern Ontario groups. In 1956 Creighton and Margaret in Fort Frances contacted Ray Connett for information and local referrals. They visited the Oakwood club in Minnesota, since the Manitoba club still had no land and Norhaven was too distant. When a Dutch couple arrived in town it seemed as though a group might form after all, but Carl and Elly became disenchanted after visiting both Oakwood and Norhaven. In 1964 Creighton gave up his efforts and sold his land.[18]

Several families in the Thunder Bay area tried to start a club during the 1950s, but it was only when a Norhaven couple, Dudley and Dorothy, arrived that locals formed the Lakehead Health Club. Members visited several of the many nearby lakes where they indulged in swimming, fishing, and nude scuba diving. Location and lack of interest caused Lakehead to fold in 1968.[19]

In 1965 a family in New Liskeard inquired about Norhaven, and, learning that they were two years too late, decided to start a club on their 500 acre farm. They provided themselves and the few members with a pool, volleyball, a rifle range, and pony rides, and optimistically promised visitors no blackflies. The Temiskaming Heliosophical Society remained largely a one-family operation, and wound down its activities in the early 1970s.[20]

Southern Ontario became the real center for club growth in the province. About 1937 a club was formed in Toronto which attracted nearly one hundred members, who enjoyed summer camp on a farm in York County. But the land was poorly screened, and neighboring parents complained that their innocent sons "were able to look through the trees and see nude bodies among the trees." Police advised the owner to install solid fencing, but the club could not afford to do so and chose to disband.[21]

Throughout the 1940s various organizers maintained a listing for Toronto in *Sunshine & Health* and continued to attract inquiries. Some of these naturists eventually joined the Sun-Air club after 1943. But locally the group remained only semi-active as a travel club. "In Toronto, there is a group, informally organized, and which has indulged in occasional outings. Its problem is, that every time it goes out, it trespasses on someone's land." Eventually the pressure of work compelled the group's leader, Jim, to pass responsibility on to another member, Bruce, in December 1948.[22]

At about the same time a new group emerged in Toronto to accommodate singles who could not get into the other one. A longtime sunbather who joined Ray Connett's *Nudist Registry* in 1947 had volunteered to act as Toronto organizer. For two years Frank, the "grand old man" of Toronto nudists, worked to bring together a group of young, single enthusiasts, who finally formed a club in October 1948. The new leader, Reg Nicholls, had also established contacts through the *Nudist Registry*, and during the summer of 1948 he invited a small nucleus of five members to use property Nicholls owned at Coe Hill, near Bancroft.[23]

On January 31, 1949, the singles group met with Bruce, the leader of the couples group, to discuss a merger on a non-quota basis. They also discussed the need for property, since Reg's land was too far away for regular use at a time when few members had cars. And they decided on a name: after briefly considering "Toron Tans Club" (TTC), they chose Sunglades.[24]

Although both groups had agreed in principle on a course of action, nothing happened for several months. *Sunny Trails* magazine noted in April 1949 that "the situation in Toronto is a bit hazy." Bruce continued to put off the day for complete merger, and Sunglades members feared he might keep his own group going and limit their prospects—particularly after one of the couples acquired land on the Trent River and invited friends to join them for sunbathing. Throughout the late 1940s and early 1950s there were persistent rumors of another large, unaffiliated club in the Toronto area. It was hard to believe that the 100 or more members of the York County club simply gave up when their first camp proved unsuitable. It also seemed puzzling that the contacts gleaned from *Sunshine & Health* listings during the 1940s mysteriously disappeared just when they were due to merge with the Sunglades Club—particularly when one of these contacts, ostensibly working for Sunglades, bought land on the Trent River and invited the organizers of the couples group for weekends. "It is quite possible that they will be pulling the local couples along with them to that property."[25]

The rumors soon turned into reports. In 1948 Boyd, a Sunglades applicant, told Reg about a landed club that existed east of Toronto and claimed that he had seen pictures of the camp where the members were nude. But Nicholls, who was not impressed with Boyd, dismissed this shadow club as "certainly not anything official, and from the description undesirable." This impression was confirmed by another Sunglades member in 1951. In 1952 a club applicant who worked at Toronto General Hospital reported that some of the doctors told him "'WE ALL' belong to a club of that kind, but not the Toronto club, one outside the city." And a few years later the secretary of the new Toronto Gymnosophical Society reported that he too had heard of "unofficial 'nudist' groups whose behavior is alien to our Naturist Movement."[26]

In the July 1949 issue of *Sunshine & Health* Reg reported on Sunglades' progress in persuading the couples group to merge with the singles and in obtaining a more convenient campground. Then, in late July, *Flash*, a notorious Toronto tabloid, shocked Sunglades with bright red front page headlines: *"LOCAL ARTIST BARED; OPERATES NUDIST COLONY."* The story itself was not all that bad, though "quite garbled and inaccurate," but the real impact came from the printing of Nicholl's full name and address.

> Well, Toronto is far more straightlaced than even Boston so this was quite a shocking story to "Toronto the good." As a result of this, Reg was dismissed from the position of head artist for the largest publishing firm in Canada.[27]

Meanwhile "pandemonium" prevailed in Sunglades as members scrambled to save their club. In the autumn they elected a new executive board, comprising several recent English immigrants: President Jimmy, Secretary Jackie, and Treasurer Ken. Jim cracked down on security, forbidding members to contact each other and refusing to send membership lists to the CSA. Whenever strangers were seen near camp members scrambled for their clothes, while Jim angrily confronted the intruders. Jim's term ended after he introduced a rule requiring husbands and wives to join together (as a singles club Sunglades had allowed married men to attend on their own). When his blushing new bride found nudism "disgusting," he was hoisted by his own petard.[28]

The group drafted a new constitution appropriate for a cooperative club and started the search for land—something that became an annual ritual. In 1950 Sunglades moved its camp west of Toronto and rented Sloan's Place, "a 50 acre cowpasture," for $300 per year. But the site was not accessible by public transportation, so the club looked around again. Members found a "beautiful park" for 1951 but couldn't afford the rent, so only in late spring did they rent "an ideal campsite which has the advantage of a small private lake," complete with its own "floating island." The 20-acre camp on the Humber River, near Nobleton, was only 35 miles from downtown Toronto, and "the natural surroundings are really very beautiful."[29]

Starting in 1950 the Sunglades Club enjoyed two years of steady growth. The new board included Ken as president and Albert "Taylor" as secretary. Both served for two years. Membership stood at 52 (26 men, 13 women, 13 children), after some people had resigned after the Flash incident. Active recruiting, tempered by careful selection, increased the figure to 72 by 1952 (20 couples, 9 single men, 4 single women, and 19 children). Members enjoyed a variety of activities including dinners, dances, and parties; art and photography classes; and indoor swimming at rented pools in the YMCA and in a Toronto apartment building until "we learned that the janitor threatened to make trouble for us." Because Sunglades was still circumspect regarding publicity it rented these facilities under the name Toronto Gymnosophical Society.[30]

In 1951 Sunglades reeled from a triple blow. When the club tried to insert advertisements in Toronto newspapers, the Globe

and the Star said "No." Only the *Telegram* accepted a brief classified ad: "Sunglades Sunbathing Club invites your application for
membership." The Toronto Police Morality Squad called the president at work to determine whether the club had its camp inside
Toronto. Ken assured them it did not, and made an appointment
to discuss the club with them. "Both the editors and police imag-
ined us as 'parading' around in front of each other." When he
invited an officer to visit the camp, "he lurched forward in his
chair in surprise," toyed with the idea briefly, then demurred. Ken
left with a police "request" not to advertise in any Toronto newspaper. "This sort of cramps the style of our publicity campaign."[31]

The most serious jolts came in the summer. First, news of the
Quetans raid in late July (see Chapter Seven) drove out "most of
the best and most desirable members." Second, in August *Flash*
came back to announce an exposé of nudist clubs based on "inside
information." (The "inside informant" was the CSA secretary-
treasurer, a Vancouver artist descended from Gainsborough.
When he "appropriated" funds "to his own use" and got caught he
wrote defamatory letters to the other board members and then
quit.) When the story broke in late August it was "the lowest
punch nudism has ever taken," and fabricated allegations that
sank "so far down into the depths of human depravity that you
would wonder that it could be written in English and still see
print." Although Connett could not resist mocking "*Phew!*" on the
"Woman's Page" of *Sunbathing for Health*, the CSA in Vancouver
decided to ignore the *Flash* article because it was manifestly "a
cheap attempt to gain circulation by pandering to the appetites of
sub-normal readers." Unfortunately the Sunglades club had to
deal with the ensuing fan mail.

> A Short time ago, I saw a piece in the *Flash* about the
> Nudists Clubs and the rest of it. I am writing to ask
> you where I can get some nudists pictures I have
> never seen any, but I can imagin what they are like I
> have heard a lot about them & I would sure love to
> have some I wonder if you could help me, I choose
> you name out of all that list drop me a line soon, as I

would like to have some nudist pictures. (Thank you) Kindly oblige.[32]

Sunglades learned the details of the *Flash* story from their own inside sources, and contacted the paper to demand that it print no names or pictures of their members. *Flash* agreed to this request, but casually informed club representatives that it had spent the entire summer of 1950 taking pictures of them at camp using tele-photo lenses. *Flash* then obtained members' names and addresses by checking license plate numbers and warned the club that if they ever obtained any evidence of "free love" at the camp the paper would publish everything. But "thanks to the good conduct of our hand-picked members we were safe." None the less, the fact that the tabloid that had nearly destroyed the club in 1949 now had names, addresses, and nude photographs kept members away from camp for the rest of the year; "most of them tell me they are through." When President Ken called a meeting in September, only six members showed up.[33]

Sunglades' anxiety over *Flash* and the other Toronto tabloids reflected the elitist image that the club cultivated. They thought they were hot stuff—better than the Granite Club—and were sure that *Flash* "would dearly love to be able to print Grant's, or the names of several of our other members holding executive posi-tions, exposing them as nudists." From the very beginning Sunglades sought out the "Cadillac" type of member. In the first year, when the club was struggling to get started, it rejected appli-cants for being "very shortsighted" or "too filthy" or "not having a pleasing personality"—all out of the desire to attract "the better class." In vain Ray Connett reminded the club that "Cadillac" members "will want Cadillac comforts and refinements."[34]

This elitism became institutionalized under Albert "Taylor," secretary from 1950 to 1952. During his first year Taylor proposed changing the club name because "'Sunglades' is still a little too revealing," and offered several alternatives: Beverly Hills Park, Monterrey Park, Santa Barbara Garden (Taylor had just returned from visiting California), Pine Valley Estates, Birch Valley

Orchards, and Tahiti Surfriders (God knows where that one came from). "Don't say that these names sound too swanky, because anything is good enough for us."[35]

In principle Sunglades elitism centered on "moral character." Taylor claimed that Sunglades had "the highest class of member of the eastern Canadian clubs," as indicated by their non-smoking, non-drinking, non-carnivoring, non-salacious conduct. "Most members prefer classical music, probably due to an education above average." And Sunglades took pride in the general appearance of their members as well—certainly when contrasted with the "large repulsive photos" from the Quetans. In practice, since "moral character" is difficult to ascertain objectively, Sunglades fell back on various material criteria which reinforced its reputation for "snobbism." Ethnic background, occupation, residence, marital status, handwriting—all were scrutinized to determine which of the many who called would be chosen. "We are continuing our strict screening policy because it has given us the best results, not in quantity but in quality."[36]

Of course, Sunglades was "strictly against racial as well as religious discrimination"—officially. But in 1949, when the first Jewish applicant showed up, caution was the by-word lest "we get a great drove of them so that the club becomes mainly Jewish. One thing that bothers me there is that if there were an accident at the club they are likely to be quick to sue." Two years later, when another Jewish couple was admitted, one member complained "how Jews have taken over in certain districts of the city." The secretary pointed out to her that all applicants should be judged as individuals, but added, "as far as taking over certain parts of the city, isn't that exactly what Roman Catholic French Canadians are doing in Quebec and in northern Ontario?" He hastily added that "some of my best friends are Roman Catholics, but they aren't ignorant at all." As for Toronto's other minorities—Chinese and Colored in particular—the former president commented that "I wouldn't want to see Sunglades overwhelmingly of any of these races or types because it would inevitably affect the club's growth."[37]

Sunglades took pride in its upper class membership: doctors, lawyers, clergymen, professors, teachers, businessmen, office workers, artists, and craftsmen. Working class folks were conspicuous by their absence—"who ever heard of a medical doctor or a business executive rubbing shoulders in social circles with ditch diggers or factory workers?" Taylor could spot—or smell—the wrong type a mile away.

> Anyone who occasionally or regularly travels through the declining districts of the city, say with the King, Queen, or Dundas streetcars, will be disgusted to notice how most men (and probably all laborers and factory workers) stink either from stale tobacco or from over-indulgence in alcoholic beverages, while the women emanate other disagreeable odors.[38]

These "zoot zooters" irresponsibly allowed their residential areas (all of Toronto south of St. Clair between Keele and Coxwell) to dilapidate into slums because they spent "all their income on liquor and other unreasonable and unhealthy luxuries," and then had the nerve to vote Communist. "Anyway, at least one usually can start breathing again when one gets on the Lawrence bus, the Forest Hill bus, or the Kingsway coach, or even the Bloor streetcar!"[39]

One of the most striking changes in membership criteria inaugurated by Taylor was the quota system for single men. The reason for the change was that Taylor suspected that "many of the male applicants are eccentrics in one way or another." "Eccentric" meant homosexual, and several applicants to Sunglades over the years were gay—causing understandable anxiety in a predominantly single male nudist club whose young camp manager "got a spanking from the gang for his birthday." When Boyd, "rather a fine looking man," applied in 1948 and asked whether he could bring along some male friends who happened to be homosexual and would "practice their 'art' in private," he was quickly turned down. Sunglades even used the homosexual angle to discredit a rival club organizer in 1952, but tempered its McCarthyite zeal because "we have a member (5 years) who was convicted, and our 'upper crust' executive knew this and still accepted him."[40]

As befit a club whose executive eschewed alcohol, tobacco, meat, and fluoride, Taylor believed that penmanship provided the window to an applicant's soul. "I can say from experience that the character of a person shows itself in his handwriting. I am sure you will have noticed yourself that a person with a sloppy handwriting is sloppy altogether." Lest this exclude all the fine doctors in the club Taylor qualified that statement: "nice handwriting can almost always be taken as a positive proof for a man's reliability;" whereas a poor pen could be excused in a rich professional. Taylor himself preferred not to test his mettle against other graphologists and avoided writing to anyone he did not like or did not want to meet.[41]

The events of 1952 broke Sunglades apart irretrievably. At the spring 1952 meeting President Ken and Secretary Albert resigned. (Actually, a "concerted effort" by other members denied Taylor reelection because of dissatisfaction with his policies and the ensuing publicity.) Since few other members stood for office Dennis, a relative newcomer, became president, Ken took over as secretary, and Terry as treasurer.[42]

In late spring, members gathered at the "floating island" property to enjoy a nice warm weekend. "We had a nice crowd, largest gathering of kids we have had out incidentally." But the owner of the land arrived and ordered the club out immediately. Sunglades had sublet the land from a farmer who had agreed to purchase the property from the owner, but this transaction had not been completed. Meanwhile the owner hired a detective to monitor the club, and when he found out that his tenants were nudists he ordered them out. By now it was too late to rent a new camp for the season, and members fell back on individual and small group outings to secluded locations or dropped out altogether.[43]

These summer events polarized opinion in Sunglades and led two executive officers and many members to resign. Dennis increasingly took over personal control of all business, easing out the other executives and prompting Reg to resign from his club in September (although his role as the new Eastern CSA Director kept him informed indirectly about Sunglades).[44]

Dennis got off to a promising start. He used club listings and articles in various magazines to boost membership to more than sixty by year's end. Along the way "it has been necessary to get rid of a few who have given us a lot of trouble . . . but I have to have a clear field in which to work if I am going to get things going." This comment set off alarm bells in the CSA, because it smacked of Gaetan Couture's strategy in the Quetans. None the less, Dennis pressed on, and by November he had purchased outright a 60-acre property near Orangeville that the club would own, not rent; he had secured provincial and municipal permits to operate a campground (Sunny Acres Camp); and he prepared to start construction in 1953. "Truely he has done more in the space of a few months here than any other exec. has accomplished in several years of work."[45]

But there were ominous portents in much of what Dennis was doing. The "NEW SUNGLADES" would be financed by shares "heavily slanted in favor of the president-and-property-owner." Most of the seventy-four members had been hand-picked by Dennis alone and lacked any knowledge of the club's previous history. And, worst of all, his business partner and principal investor was "an undesirable character" whom Reg and others accused of wife swapping, picture trading, and hosting nude house parties. At the first meeting of the "happy" new members in February 1953, the twenty-seven present voted to hand over all control of the club to Dennis and Glenn to "run the club this year as WE see fit." That was the last official communication from Sunglades; sometime during 1953 Dennis quietly made off with the club land, assets, and records, leaving the "happy" members to fend for themselves.[46] No one from the club went after him.

> I have been warned however that Dennis here has sufficient connection with personnel of the local police and other business connections to make it "hot" for anyone here who might show opposition to him.[47]

CHAPTER SIX

Ontario Outdoors

Within a year after the demise of the Sunglades Club in 1953 left a momentary void in southern Ontario, a whole new phase of organization and growth would commence which continues today. SAFL/ Norhaven and Sunglades provided many Ontarians with club experience, and some of these nudists went on to form their own clubs. They were joined in the mid-1950s by an influx of British and European immigrants with naturist experience. Together Canadians and New Canadians soon established half a dozen major clubs throughout Ontario, and these clubs in turn spun off another set of clubs in the 1960s, with more to follow. Affluence, the growing popularity of summertime retreats in "cottage country," and the newly-awakened mass interest in the great outdoors, especially on summer vacations, contributed to an increasing desire to get back to nature that made nudism more popular than before.

Glen Echo, also known as Toronto Gymnosophical Society, emerged from the residue of Sunglades members left after their president absconded with the assets in 1953. Old magazine listings continued to bring in new applicants, mostly British and German immigrants, who joined with the remaining Sungladers on 28 February 1954 to form the Toronto Gymnosophical Society as a new beginning. Eight couples and two singles attended the first TGS meeting, which elected the first executive board.[1]

There now commenced an agonizingly long search for land. The on-again, off-again efforts discouraged many members who either dropped out or moved closer to the Niagara club, which offered generous terms to the Toronto group until it could find land. A few were briefly tempted to join Count Eberhard, a German immigrant and engineer who launched his own trial balloon, the Sunshine Club, but soon ran out of hot air.[2]

Then a small miracle happened. While the TGS executive was negotiating futilely with a variety of farmers and real estate agents, another member couple, Eddy and Mary Todorowsky, was quietly and systematically conducting their own search for land. Although both came from Saskatchewan, they had met in Toronto and had visited local beaches for clandestine skinnydips. They married in 1949, and while they were on honeymoon at Wasaga Beach, Eddy spotted *Sunbathing for Health* on a newsstand (it was still not available in Toronto) and this introduced him to organized nudism. They later joined the Toronto club.[3]

In 1954 the Todorowskys visited several American clubs, and this whetted their desire for a club in Toronto. In June 1955 they targeted a 100 acre tract of woodland due north of Toronto, and drove out to inspect the site on the July holiday. Although they had started by searching for their own family farm, the "peace and quietness in this valley" so entranced them that Eddy agreed to make it available for club use. Todorowsky took possession of the land two weeks later, and Glen Echo was born.[4]

On 11 September 1955, fifteen families and five single members gathered at Glen Echo to hold the first General Meeting in their new home. Everyone could see the potential of the abandoned lumber camp, with its central valley and weed-infested creek gurgling somewhere under the brush, all surrounded by wooded hills. The club secretary, Bill, recognized the site after his own explorations. "Eddy, by devoted labor, had brush cleared and grass mowed, so that we were able to drive right in, to a lovely parkland rolling down to the creek" (which had been uncovered at last). At the meeting, owners and members agreed on the "plan of operation" and the "scheme for progressive development." Briefly, it was understood that Eddy and Mary owned the land and were responsible for all development there. In return for making this land available as "a beautiful and permanent place for nudism," TGS agreed to remit all membership and ground fees, other than modest office expenses, to the landowners, who were also entitled to all cabin and campsite rents.[5] Because of the demands on all members to help develop the club, this "understanding" was not formalized in a written agreement until 1962.

The centerpiece of the camp was a large pool created by bull-dozing the river bed and damming the water to create a pond 200 feet long and 4 feet deep. The first pool was ready by 1956, then enlarged in 1958 and again two years later on a grander scale, becoming the two-acre Lake Echo, complete with its own little island. By this time the club also had a children's wading pool. Further amenities included volleyball courts, washrooms and showers, and motel units.[6] TGS maintained members' interest during the long winter months by hosting social events such as pot luck dinners, parties, and dances in members' homes or in rented halls, and by arranging indoor recreation activities like swimming in a rooftop pool in downtown Toronto and volleyball at the Oakville-Trafalgar High School.[7]

By 1960 the effort to improve the grounds had largely succeeded. Glen Echo was well established as a campground, but TGS board members lacked the determination to push for further development at a time when a new generation of full-service resort clubs made its appearance in the United States and Canada. "While there is still much to be done, the general appearance and amenities are now thoroughly satisfactory and this drive has been lost." The reluctance of TGS to increase fees or membership numbers meant that efforts by the owner-manager to undertake developments and improvements were financed on a hand-to-mouth basis. At the annual general meeting on 17 July 1967, Eddy informed members that "Glen Echo is not paying its way," and asked for full control over club operations: in other words, a straightforward proprietary operation, without the awkward intermediary of a "society" whose executive lacked a stake in the camp. The written agreement between the owner and TGS, signed only five years earlier, could be terminated at any time by mutual consent (Article 12), and members "agreed to this in a free vote."[8]

This decision and the subsequent fee increase allowed Todorowsky to begin a new phase of construction, starting with the all-year clubhouse in 1973. The central feature was a 25-by-50 foot heated indoor swimming pool, accompanied by sauna, whirlpool, and indoor washrooms. Upstairs he installed a large lounge with pool and ping-pong tables, snackbar, and office space. In 1979 a visiting ASA officer wrote that "TGS was a beautiful club and a real nudist atmosphere," and so it has remained, as a *Toronto Sun* reporter found in 1995, on the fortieth anniversary of Glen Echo.

> Everywhere you turn on this breathtakingly beautiful 100 acre paradise are bronzed, healthy, naked people. Young and old, supple or chunky, male and female, they all carry on in their favorite summer activities *au naturel* and, seemingly, without a care in the world.[9]

Over the years several short-lived clubs spun off from Glen Echo because of the resistance of other individualists to a determined proprietor and the desire to be their own boss and run a club their own way. The Society of Health (Bolton), Toronto Health and Sun Club (Sandford), and Cedar Valley (Orono) all came and went. The only successful breakaway club was Toronto Helios, near Sharon north of Newmarket, but after 15 years it too turned textile. (The campground has now returned to nudism under new management.)[10]

In the middle of the Golden Horseshoe, Hamilton saw several early attempts at club formation. In 1949 two Hamilton men stepped forward to act as group leaders. Butch, a Sunglades member recommended by Reg Nichols, contacted the CSA. But his bid for CSA recognition failed when the Quetans reported on his visit to Montreal. Though fluently bilingual, and "a really very beautiful specimen of manhood," he seemed too beautiful to the Quetans, who concluded that "he must be some kind of pansy."[11]

In 1951 the CSA recognized Jim, a Hamiltonian with British club experience, as the district organizer, but soon found that he lacked "organizing ability." But when someone with organizing ability arrived in town, he became associated with questionable applicants and outside interests that were incompatible with CSA interests and policies. Jack, newly arrived from Saskatchewan (where he had also acted as CSA organizer), quickly attracted ten couples, bought some land, and opened camp in summer 1952, just when Sunglades lost its campground. After obtaining additional evidence, the CSA dismissed Jack as official group leader.[12]

In 1951 a naturist couple in the Niagara peninsula, who belonged to the CSA and had experience of Norhaven and Halcyon (a club in Pennsylvania), approached the CSA "in hopes a group may be formed in the Niagara District." Two years later a local farmer and lifelong naturist with access to land contacted the Niagara Group to offer help "with some of the work in preparing a camp here at Welland." In August these enthusiasts acquired land north of Fonthill and created the Niagara Gymnosophical Society (NGS). The camp opened on 23 May 1954. The Sunglades club in Toronto had folded, so many Toronto nudists were willing to travel to Niagara in order to have a club.[13]

NGS was listed in *Sunshine & Health* and *Sunbathing for Health* and in 1954 attracted a new German immigrant, Karl Ruehle, who was getting frustrated with the delays at the Toronto club and now "left the Toronto group . . . in an unkind manner." Ruehle threw himself into the hard work of turning a wooded farm lot into an attractive nudist camp. "I don't know anyone who could have made so many improvements on a campsite in such a short time." Mel, the original organizer, backed out for family reasons, and NGS gave Karl complete control to develop the club along CSA guidelines.[14]

Sun Valley Gardens (SVG) started the 1954 season with 25 acres of wooded farmland and eighteen adult members. Another seventy people joined as work progressed. "Everywhere you see the product of industry and of imagination." In 1956 the 80-foot kidney-shaped swimming pool was completed, and would long remain the centerpiece of the club. Then another 14 acres was acquired, and Ruehle promoted Sun Valley Heights—a nudist subdivision where people could "live a most natural life all year 'round." Another project, the Sun Valley Health and Recreation Club, would contribute to the club's later split with the CSA.[15]

By this time Sun Valley had more than 300 members, and was "undoubtedly Canada's largest and finest club." The phenomenal growth stemmed from Ruehle's active, indeed aggressive publicity campaign. He distributed press releases, bought paid advertising, and appeared on talk shows and TV programs such as the "Claim to Fame" show on CHCH Hamilton where he won a wristwatch because no guessed that there was a nudist camp proprietor in darkest Ontario.[16]

Ruehle's most successful publicity stunts were the open house days that he started in 1956. In early May he invited the press out to discuss his plans for the event, and *Toronto Telegram* reporters Ron Collister and Ian Paterson duly wrote about "a warm naked welcome," although the lone reporter for the tabloid *Hush* explained that the *Telegram* sent two men so that one could keep an eye on the other, and cautioned Ron Collister against greeting nude young ladies with an overly enthusiastic "Wowie!"[17]

Sixty local officials received invitations to visit camp on 24 June 1956. Although only one lonely deputy reeve showed up, he was accompanied by an army of thirty reporters and photographers who provided "longer and more detailed stories than we have ever had in the West." The day before the nude open house the general public was invited to visit the club while members were dressed "in order not to offend anyone not accustomed to our way of living." Five hundred people toured the camp, and more than 100 inquired about membership and a return visit under normal conditions.[18]

In 1959, Ruehle opened Sun Valley Gardens to the general public on Saturday, May 30, while members were nude. Over 1,000 visitors signed affidavits that "at no time and in no way will we object to—or feel offended by—the nudity and activities of the people whom we see or meet." Many were not only not offended, but joined in nude activities, and nearly 100 joined the club. There was full media coverage from Toronto and Buffalo newspapers and the Canadian Broadcasting Corporation. The event confirmed Sun Valley as "the largest and certainly the most progressive club in all of Canada." It also split the club apart.[19]

By 1959 Sun Valley Gardens was "not well known for the democratic spirit of its leaders." Members and visitors alike regarded Ruehle as autocratic and tight-fisted. He objected when people moved camp furniture, even if only to place a chair or picnic table in the shade. He interrupted games and competitions if they lasted longer than his schedule allowed. He closely monitored new couples in their tents. Many saw him as a "boot stomping Prussian."[20]

For years members had been leaving Sun Valley to form new clubs. London Sun Club, Sunshine Ranch, Sunny Glades, Sunny Acres, Ponderosa, and Lilly Valley all had their origin in SVG alumni. In most cases Karl wished them well, and stayed in touch. Only one effort did he thwart, an attempt by a former member to set up a rival camp virtually across the street. But the farmer whose land was up for lease, and who knew Karl well, reneged on the deal after Ruehle spoke with him.[21]

In later years Ruehle moderated his policy and his behavior in response to the continuing defection of Canadians to new clubs in Ontario and the emergence of nudist clubs in New York State— home to half of his members—once that state relaxed its anti-nudity laws. In fact Ruehle, who started out advocating European-style naturism over American-style nudity, soon settled into a "very mellow" practice of nudism. By the 1970s Sun Valley Gardens admitted singles as well as couples regardless of whether they were divorced, separated, or married with a reluctant spouse. Body contact and even sex were permitted, if not encouraged. Moreover, Sun Valley offered a health club with communal bathing and massage; a social club for dances and parties; and a camera club with nude models in exclusive photo sessions and confidential photo-developing services.[22]

Despite all the attractions, membership continued to decline. In 1974, the twentieth anniversary, only one other original member remained (Ken, also from Sunglades). Although new members continued to drop by, not enough stayed to keep the club going. In 1982 Ruehle put Sun Valley up for sale. When no satisfactory offers came in, he converted the camp into a conventional RV park.[23]

In 1959 disgruntled members of Sun Valley Gardens left the club to reestablish the Niagara Gymnosophical Society on a more democratic basis as a cooperative club. After trying out several names (Sunhaven, Norwood), they eventually settled on the Olympus Health and Recreation Club, at a meeting held in Buffalo on 23 April 1960. At this time Olympus comprised twenty-six adults and ten children. The club acquired land east of Dunnville, Ontario, for a new camp to be called Sandy Acres. Peggy Parkes, *grande dame* of the club, scored several publicity coups by appearing on Hamilton radio and TV programs during the 1960s on behalf of Olympus and the Eastern Canadian Sunbathing Association (ECSA). But in the early sixties "a couple of troublemakers" upset club life, and it did not recover momentum until 1962 when the new "Olympian Herald" announced "the rebirth of Olympus." The club hosted ECSA conventions in 1963 and 1965, then went through another reorganization before folding for good in 1973.[24]

Lilly Valley opened in 1963. Ludwig and Lilly Mueller brought their European nudist experience with them, but found Kamloops unsympathetic to even a nude baby on the beach. When they moved to Ontario they joined Sun Valley Gardens. Eventually, like many other members of that club, they got the idea that "one of these days we will have our sun club." In July 1963, they opened Lilly Valley in Fort Erie as "a club to create a healthy body through a healthy mind by recreation, air, and sunbathing." On 52 acres they offered a small, family-oriented "home away from home."

Facilities include one of the first heated indoor swimming pools at a Canadian nudist club, a sauna and hot tub, and the usual outdoor games of volleyball, badminton, and horseshoes.[25]

For a time Lilly Valley was occasionally confused with the By-Sun Club—also a defector from Sun Valley—which set up in 1965 just across the highway from Lilly Valley, but never developed. "The whole thing looks like a junkyard and is wide open to the curious eye." The crude screening created at By-Sun by bulldozing mounds of dirt created "an abominable eyesore" that provoked many local complaints and triggered an attempt by the Ridgeway-Bertie Township Council to enact a by-law against nudist camps. The Muellers and the ECSA protested this action, even though it was not retroactive, lest it "create the habit of some sex maniacs coming to our gate and asking for membership."[26]

Lilly Valley prided itself on its policy of "complete nudity at all times" and on maintaining a strict gender balance by requiring single men to bring female partners to the club. Lilly Valley also aimed to promote "families in harmony with nature," and in 1991 the club hosted Juniorfest, a day of fun and games intended to demonstrate that nudism is for kids and not just for adults. But at times the heavy emphasis on family togetherness backfired, as when some visiting families felt they were wrongly labelled as "swingers" and the ECSA was compelled to investigate. Nonetheless, Lilly Valley remained popular with its fifty-odd members, and celebrated its thirtieth anniversary with month-long festivities during July 1993. Lilly died in 1994, and Ludwig in 1995. The club grounds were sold in 1999.[27]

In 1961 John and Irene Pries opened Sunny Acres Nature Park near Rockwood, Ontario. They had prior experience on the island of Sylt in Germany and at Sun Valley Gardens. In 1960 they purchased 10 acres of land with a spring-fed pond, which they harnessed to supply the swimming pool. The club was mainly a family operation open to friends. But the area was developing rapidly with new housing, and so the Pries family found a larger 42-acre site nearby in 1969. Here the "main drawing point" was a 1 1/2 acre artificial lake with a 1000 foot sand beach, surrounded by "towering cedars" providing a "fairy forest setting." Unfortunately, drainage problems emptied the lake and it proved impractical to re-do the whole job. The family moved back to its first home, and the club remained limited to a few friends.[28]

In 1962 two German-Canadian couples, related by marriage and former members of Sun Valley Gardens, bought 100 acres of wooded land near Strabane, north of Hamilton, and began building the Ponderosa Nature Park. Development was carefully planned around a large clubhouse and a giant L-shaped swimming pool blasted out of bedrock and holding "a million litres of sparkling water." The camp opened in 1964, the pool was completed in 1965, and Ponderosa hosted its first ECSA convention in 1966 with more preparation than most clubs. "An amazing amount of good work has been done. Also, the planning and design of the whole project were very pleasing to us."[29]

The ECSA saw one fly in the ointment. Although "we like these people and the attitude to nudism and naturism which they expressed," there were suspicions about a lax policy on alcohol. More than one board member came to ECSA convention determined to "kick Ponderosa out of the association." After due deliberation (without anyone from Ponderosa present) the board voted "that Ponderosa Nature Park should not be associated with ECSA at this time because of Ponderosa's different philosophy and practice respecting alcoholic beverages." Later, when the board met with the owners, both sides worked out a "remarkably amicable agreement" whereby Ponderosa would clarify its "philosophy and practice" and the ECSA would "leave it to 'the grapevine'" to determine whether the new policy was successful. In fact, Ontario changed its law regarding alcohol in campgrounds at this time, while the ASA was moving to reconsider its policies as well.[30]

During the 1960s and 1970s Ponderosa attracted a steady stream of new members, some of them from Sun Valley Gardens, some from New York State, most from the Golden Horseshoe area of Southern Ontario. As membership increased, it added more facilities. In 1979 the clubhouse underwent remodelling to accommodate a heated indoor pool, sauna, and whirlpool. Then in 1987 the Albrechts sold the club to New Country Investors, a group that included Herbert Hofmann, formerly a member of Four Seasons. The Albrechts separated a 10 acre plot for their retirement home, leaving the club with 90 acres, 40 of which are protected conservation marsh and home to wildlife, which can be seen by members walking the three nature trails. Present outdoor facilities include volleyball on four courts, tennis, basketball, shuffleboard, baseball, a children's playground, and golf on a regulation par-3 69-yard pitching green complete with sand trap and water hazard. Special events include volleyball, golf, and tennis tournaments, and a childrens' day competition. Ponderosa members also participate in inter-club volleyball competitions, including the Superbowl at White Thorn Lodge in Pennsylvania. In 2002 the club changed hands once again as longtime members Lee and Brad took over the operation and launched a series of improvements.[31]

The Four Seasons Nature Park was founded in 1969 by Hans and Lisa Stein, former members of Sun Valley Gardens and former partners in Ponderosa. In 1968, seeking their own club to be run their own way—particularly with year-round operations to compensate for the short Canadian outdoor season—they purchased a 35-acre homesite off Highway 6 north of Hamilton. Four Seasons opened in January 1969. A clubhouse was built around the existing swimming pool, converting it to indoor use. And in a unique touch, the pool also doubles as the club's dance floor, once an 8 ton platform is lowered from the ceiling; no wasted space here.[32]

The two-part Alpine-style clubhouse includes a lavish upstairs gym, motel rooms, a sauna and whirlpool, and a newly remodelled nightclub complex, Scandals. The clubhouse, nightclub, and gazebo all have full service bars. Other facilities include volleyball and tennis courts, which were home to the First Canadian Nudist Volleyball Open Tournament in 1994. For its own Nudist Volleyball Open Tournaments the club uses professional referees. What the Eastern Sunbathing Association reported in 1970 is still true today: "the grounds and huge clubhouse are first class at Four Seasons, better than most Holiday Inns—just beautiful."[33]

Four Seasons gained a giant lead over all other Canadian nudist clubs with its tremendously successful Miss Nude World contests. All nudists complain about the disparity in the extent of social nudism in Europe and in North America, but the Steins decided to do something about it. "We wanted to have nudism talked about, to prompt people to visit a nudist camp." While other clubs had hosted nude open house events for the public, Four Seasons staged an event that would draw even larger crowds, on the gamble that many would decide to join after seeing a club in a non-threatening, no-pressure situation.[34]

In 1970, the first year the contest was held, twelve contestants vied for the title; Rhonda Stallan from Glen Echo was chosen after careful scrutiny from a panel of distinguished judges including Toronto radio broadcaster Gordon Sinclair (making his own fashion statement in a fine kilt). Media coverage was so extensive that it preempted reports about Prime Minister Trudeau's attendance at the reopening of the Welland Canal on the same weekend. The next year eighteen contestants competed in late July during 90°F weather that prompted most of the audience to undress. Rosemarie Hess from the Domaine Naturiste du Québec won that year. 1972 was a very successful year, perhaps the best in the series. 5,000 people attended and police turned away another 5000 when the back-up on Highway 6 topped 5 miles. Twenty-nine contestants entered, and Jocelyne Lepine from the Paradis Terrestre club in Quebec was the winner. It was a true spectacle, and the media had fun like everyone else.[35]

By 1976 the Miss Nude World contest had become too large for the Four Seasons club to host, and the event moved off-site to public hotels and convention centers, starting at the El Morocco Club and ending at the Milgrove Speedway. The contest lost much of its appeal to contestants and nudists because "it's not within the environment of what the original idea was." Rather than risk further adverse publicity Lisa Stein, who retains legal control of the Miss

Nude World title, stopped the contests completely. Four Seasons continues to hold its own in-house contests for members, including Olympic and Junior Olympic competitions, Miss Four Seasons, and Mr Nude World—won in 1977 by "Dy-no-mite Bob"— "he's so skinny that when he stood sideways the judges almost missed him."[36]

On Victoria Day weekend 1994, Four Seasons celebrated its silver anniversary as "Canada's premier naturist resort." Five hundred members and guests joined in tribute to the Stein family for their "dedication, sacrifice, hard and on-going work, and a willingness to be always 'on'." But after more than forty years of development and expansion the Stein family had enough and put the club up for sale in 2002.[37]

In 1955 some members of Sun Valley Gardens decided to organize the London Sun Club. Later that year the founders, Ed and Jean, bought a 45-acre site to develop as a campground, which became Sun-Mor Park, located 16 miles southeast of London near Harrietsville. The founders owned the land and leased it to the club. Members developed a volleyball court, children's playground, and swimming pool.[38]

In 1957 Sun-Mor Park hosted the CSA Eastern convention, and in 1959 they invited prospective members on Visitors Day. In 1960 they hosted the first ECSA convention. Then in 1962 the founding family sold the camp to a group of nine members who set about improving operations, developing a library, and printing a club newsletter, *Sun Mor News*. But some members of the consortium decided that they could do things better and tried to seize control. This prompted others to set out on their own. In October 1964, the club held a meeting to close up shop and sell the land for a textile campground.[39]

Ted and Pam Lisiecki had been members of the London Sun Club since 1955 and were part of the consortium that bought the land from Ed and Jean in 1962. By 1965 it was clear that the old club was finished, so some of the members met with the Lisieckis to create the Summerset Travel Club, a non-landed group. In 1966 Ted bought the London Sun Club property from himself and the other eight owners. The London Summerset Club developed all the usual amenities, and arranged indoor winter games at Sir Adam Beck and Wheable schools in London and at the South Dorchester school.[40]

Summerset had considerable success with special events. In 1971 the club held its first nude open house to "acquaint the general public with the values and benefits of nudism." The event was more popular with the visitors—one of whom admitted "I feel embarrassed walking around with clothes on"—than with some members who stayed dressed for the occasion. In 1972 members staged the nudist play *Barely Proper* for public audiences. Then in 1973 Summerset scored its biggest coup with the Miss Nude Ontario competition on 22 July. Eight contestants competed in front of 1800 visitors attracted by extensive advertising. People who missed the show could watch it on CFPL London, which provided coverage from ground level and helicopter. The contest was repeated in 1974 and 1975, but by this time these contests had outlived their usefulness.[41]

By the mid-1970s Summerset started losing members. In 1972 a small group broke away out of "dissatisfaction with the facilities and management of that club" to form the London Naturist Travel Club. Others went to nearby landed clubs, particularly Ponderosa and Four Seasons, which Summerset could not match in terms of facilities. In 1978 the club ceased operation.[42]

Stan Wortner grew up on a farm in southwest Ontario, where he acquired a longing for trees and an interest in nudism courtesy of *Sunbathing for Health* magazine, which he bought at a pool hall in Chatham. In the mid-1950s he and his wife, Pearl, visited Sun Valley Gardens. As he saw what to do and what not to do in running a camp, he started planning for his own venture. In 1959 he bought 94 acres of wooded land that had many rare hardwood trees and various "sunny glades" that gave the club its name. "The policy of this proprietary camp was to preserve as much of the basic contour and naturalness of the land as possible." In laying out the club with minimal environmental damage, the Wortners uncovered a number of ancient native arrowheads, which are carefully preserved in the clubhouse.[43]

In March 1961 Sunny Glades contacted the ASA regarding "affiliation with a national organization." Wortner had intended to "go it alone," but because of his projected cross-border membership he decided to work with the National Nudist Council because of its "simplicity of procedure, absence of red tape and politics," but when it offered little practical assistance he approached the ASA—gingerly. The executive director assured the club, somewhat disingenuously, that ASA's red tape was "greatly exaggerated" and that Sunny Glades could remain exclusively proprietary. Sunny Glades eventually joined the ECSA and hosted its 1962 convention, complete with extensive coverage from CFPL-TV, which was "very daring in showing full view pictures of our new Queen, Prince, and Princess," along with a volleyball game and other camp scenes. The film itself became the topic of discussion on London radio talk shows for several days.[44]

Development of the club proceeded carefully. After installing an access road, washrooms, games courts, and in-ground pool (with a unique plastic roof that speeds up heating in the spring and extends the season into the autumn), Sunny Glades received its Ontario first-class campground license and started to advertise in Chatham, Sarnia, Windsor and London. Public relations were not neglected, either: a talk on nudism before the Thamesville Rotary Club "enlightened the intelligentsia," and a casual one-hour chat with the Ontario Provincial Police brought the assurance that "we'll be there if you need us." Later, when the Wortner's daughter graduated from high school, a party was held for the class at camp, and three classmates eventually joined the club.[45]

About 1970 Stan resigned from his outside job to work full time at camp. A huge clubhouse was built by hand during the 1970s from two derelict barns and other materials, including enough bricks for a wall-to-wall fireplace. A sauna and whirlpool (which he found to be "more complex than the swimming pool") were added indoors; and a five-hole golf course and pond were added outdoors. Wortner also helped meet expenses by selling Christmas trees and maple syrup.[46]

When the club opened, many of the members were from Michigan. But over the years the proportion of Canadians to Americans has risen to more than four to one. Sunny Glades has attracted fall-out members from the London Sun Club, Summerset, and Holiday Valley, and new-generation members from southwestern Ontario. It has about 200 members, many of whom have year-round trailers. Since 1995 members have participated in the Bothwell summer parade.[47]

In 1974 Fred and Nellie Lammers, members of the Ponderosa Club since 1969, decided to venture out on their own. They purchased 100 acres of rolling wooded land west of London and started to develop the Holiday Valley Nature Resort. They put in a road, dug a swimming pool, installed hydro, located a water supply with the help of a diviner (a technique also employed at East Haven), and put up the prefabricated clubhouse in three weeks. On Saturday, 29 June, the Lammers held open house for area residents; they were "surprised to see so many local couples come out." On Sunday and Monday of this holiday weekend the club opened for nudism.[48]

Facilities at Holiday Valley included a multi-level clubhouse with a well-stocked (and heavily promoted) bar, a large in-ground swimming pool, games courts for volleyball, badminton, basketball, horseshoes, archery, and mini-golf; a sauna; and a children's petting zoo with chickens, ducks, and rabbits. "The fowl are rather stand-offish, but the rabbits are very friendly." In winter the club offered snowmobiling, cross-country skiing, toboggan rides, and skating, although most members preferred warmer locations and stayed away.[49]

Periodically the owners reminded members that the club was primarily a business, which they (the members) had to subsidize, particularly the clubhouse and bar. The club allowed members to run a tab and encouraged non-members to sign a blank credit card slip. In 1978 dues went up. In 1979 Holiday Valley joined the ASA because it seemed the easiest way to attract new visitors. However, ASA affiliation could provide only a long-term solution, and meantime the short-term expenses continued to mount. At the end of the summer the club blamed the ASA and the members for not providing sufficient profit and closed the club, turning it into a conventional campground.[50]

In 1956 Glen and June Eaton left Sun Valley Gardens to start the Riverside Sun Club in Grey County. Eaton, a war veteran, pilot, and barn painter, bought a 100-acre wooded farm north of Durham on the Styx River, near Louise Lake. The Bentinck township council reluctantly accepted Sunshine Ranch. The camp offered the usual camping, swimming, fishing, volleyball, badminton, ping pong, and horseshoes, along with Eaton's airplane rides over the Grey-Bruce area. (When Eaton attended the CSA Eastern Division convention at Glen Echo in 1958 he "caused more consternation to the Ontario Provincial Police and local inhabitants than the convention" by buzzing the area before landing in a nearby field.) In 1959 Sunshine Ranch hosted a convention in July. But Eaton was one of many club owners who became dissatisfied with nudist politics and gave up his affiliation with the ECSA/ASA, while his increasing business responsibilities drew him away from club activities. Membership gradually fell off, particularly when a new camp opened virtually next door. Eaton closed Sunshine Ranch in 1962.[51]

In 1960 Ralph left Sunshine Ranch to form the Cedarwood Naturist Park, also on the Styx River. Cedarwood had hundreds of acres of "rolling fields" and "deep cedar forest" for rustic camping. Ralph was committed to "old-fashioned naturism. Our membership is restricted to a number of families who enjoy it so, enjoy each other's company, respect each other's need for quiet, and respect the need of nature for love and care." This dedication attracted members from Sunshine Ranch and from other clubs who appreciated the peaceful natural surroundings. In 1973, when the ECSA transformed itself into the Canadian Nudist Confederation (CNC), some members of Cedarwood joined the CNC as the Cedarwood Naturist Society, while unaffiliated members and visitors used Cedarwood Naturist Park—an arrangement reminiscent of Karl Ruehle's NGS/SVG operation in Welland. Cedarwood avoided commercial advertising because the contacts "were of poor caliber. It seems that such publicity is no use for attracting the kind of people we want in this rather out of the way location." Cedarwood remained a restful haven for its thirty member families until it closed in 1983.[52]

In 1955 a European couple living in Peterborough contacted Ray Connett "to start the organizational framework of a future club." Together with some local and Toronto-area friends, they went on outings in the Kawarthas, "one of the most beautiful holiday playgrounds of Ontario." They enjoyed "all forms of outdoor living in the nude" on weekend treks to "out of the way spots."[53]

In 1956 two couples bought a 50-acre wooded farm at Upsley, near Peterborough, and established the Peterborough Sun Club at Sunnybrae Ranch. They made cautious contact with the *Peterborough Examiner* and the OPP. But this policy backfired when two families from the Toronto club visited Peterborough without prior arrangement and inquired locally about the club. The police obligingly called the owner at work, and the paper got ahold of the story. The result was that "all day Sunday there was a stream of cars passing in the vicinity of the club." Because of this incident the club suspended operations until they could find a more secluded location.[54]

In 1959 two member couples at Sunnybrae bought 100 acres near Norwood, which brought with it a new set of problems: porcupines ate the plywood faster than members could build cabins, and beavers kept remodelling dams in the river before usable pools could be created. The dozen or so members enjoyed camp until 1961, when the founder sold the land and moved to Toronto. The remaining members gradually lost interest or joined other clubs. Sunnybrae folded officially in 1962.[55]

In Kingston the first CSA contacts were Arthur and Jean, stationed at the Royal Military College. They were members of Norhaven; Art was vice-president of the club. Both had visited ASA headquarters at Sunshine Park in May's Landing, New Jersey. On this basis the CSA encouraged them to act as group leaders for the Kingston area. Not surprisingly, many of their contacts were military personnel; equally unsurprising, Art was transferred away in 1951 and Kingston was left on its own for the rest of the decade.[56]

In 1959 Hans and Maria Behrmann acquired a 165-acre woodlot surrounding Davis Lake, laying the foundation for Lakesun, the "crown jewel" of Ontario clubs. The Behrmanns had arrived in Canada in 1951, one of the few nudists of German/Austrian background to learn of nudism *after* reaching Canada (on a radio program in Hamilton in 1956). Behrmann visited Sun Valley Gardens and Norhaven, where he enjoyed waterskiing so much that this determined the kind of club that he wanted for himself.[57]

Geology also determined the way Lakesun would be built: with lots of dynamite to level the rocky surface. For many years Behrmann spent all his spare time at camp "hacking a club out of bare rock and bush, practically single-handed." He laboriously prepared a clubhouse, showers, games courts, and camping sites, all designed to blend into this "Garden of Eden in the Canadian woodlands." But it is the lake that remains the centerpiece. Davis Lake is quite shallow, so it warms quickly, making swimming, sailing, windsurfing, and canoeing very popular. Cliffs along one shore of the lake provide panoramic vistas and a 20-foot diving platform for the brave lad featured in the *Canada Naturally* video. Waterskiing also used to be popular, and Behrmann frequently ran skiers around the lake with his speedboat, until he learned that the motorboat disrupted the nesting habits of the loons that visited the lake. When the boating stopped, the loons moved back and became full-time members of the club.[58]

Lakesun is "a rare retreat of pristine beauty," and the owner is determined to keep it that way, with regulations preserving the flora and fauna. Behrmann believes that "we, as human beings are intruders and the ever-increasing population of our kind is putting hard pressure on our fellow creatures who, apart from mosquitoes, make our stay much more pleasant and enjoyable in the great outdoors." Club members appreciate the effort and determination to preserve the natural character of Lakesun. "It is a family-oriented naturist resort and its tranquil beauty is yet to be surpassed by any camp we have ever visited."[59]

At times, however, the owner's concern for nature has led to over-regulation of the "human intruders." Lakesun acquired a unique reputation in the 1960s with its rules "against everything but deep breathing." Lakesun deplored "permissive society," "revolting unnatural sex," and "weird looking" men with long hair.

Actually, the club simply found itself out of step as it clung to ASA standards—though not to the ASA—at a time when the "culture shock" of the 1960s affected all nudist clubs. The bane of social nudism, in Behrmann's view, was alcohol: "anyone with even a breath of this troublesome stuff in camp will be asked to leave—for good."[60]

What was good for Lakesun, moreover, was good for everyone else. Lakesun attempted to impose its morality on other clubs by banning visitors from clubs that allowed alcohol, and by expelling visitors who broke Lakesun rules. This "fanaticism" discouraged visits by people who shared his standards but not his policies. "We really are very fond of Hans and Maria, and had a wonderful time at Lakesun as ever, but we have to admit that Hans' over-enthusiasm does make the atmosphere there too tense for our complete comfort." Although Behrmann reiterated his opposition to alcohol as late as 1974, he relaxed his stance shortly afterwards, influenced perhaps by the moderating influence of otherwise-respectable visitors, perhaps to his own observations at the Lake Como Club in Florida where he winters. Other moralistic policies have also changed, although the transition was accompanied by a wholesale purge of malcontents in the late seventies. The more relaxed ambience makes Lakesun one of the most popular rustic camps for visitors today.

> We have been to many other fine camps in the U.S. and Canada, but the natural beauty of this club offers peace of mind with relaxation and fun, which is truly enjoyable.[61]

In the Ottawa area one of the couples associated with Max Wertheim in Montreal during his search for land in 1958 (see Chapter Eight) preferred a large farm that the group located south of Ottawa near Burritts Rapids. Frank and Marlies had visited Sun Valley Gardens in 1957, and Karl Ruehle referred them to Max. But when they saw the 400-acre spread they quit the East Haven group and gathered several other Ottawa-area couples together in a new club, SilvaSun. Three members—Frank, George, and Gerry—bought the land and made it available to members for club use in exchange for their paying property taxes. Christmas-tree sales were supposed to finance development, but no one except the three owners pursued this task. In fact, the lack of a lease agreement plagued the club throughout its history, since members hesitated to contribute money or work for the benefit of three absentee landowners (Frank stayed away after members ignored the small pool he built single-handedly and set up a larger one, and business kept the other two in Ottawa so often that when one showed up unannounced the manager chased him away).[62]

In 1968 SilvaSun incorporated as a society, and the owners agreed to a twenty-year lease. The club then offered to host the next ECSA convention, but two of the owners reneged on the lease at the last moment and the club had to rescind their agreement. Despite these problems, members did have a number of facilities to enjoy over the years, both at camp and in rented winter pools and saunas. One item that they sorely missed was a clubhouse after the first one burned in 1965. Members became discouraged by a wave of vandalism in the 1970s, and separatism accentuated differences between anglophone and francophone members at this time. But in the end it was the lack of a lease, and discord among the three owners, that doomed the club. Over the years Frank bought out George, then Gerald, and finally in the early in the 1980s he unceremoniously evicted the last resident member. By this time other members had dropped out, or had joined East Haven, taking the club back full circle.[63]

$\mathcal{T}$rouble in $\mathcal{P}$aradise

The many lakes, rivers, and wooded mountains of the Belle Province encouraged Quebecers to share in the Canadian tradition of skinny-dipping and sunbathing. But the postwar development of social nudism in Quebec was hindered by the Roman Catholic Church and its political ally, Premier Maurice Duplessis. In his "Sunny Trails" column in 1948 Ray Connett called Quebec the "question mark in Canadian nudism." Although several early clubs appeared in Quebec during the 1940s, most faded quickly. Those that would not fade were forcibly suppressed. "We must be very careful because Quebec is so severe." The best expedient seemed to be the pattern followed by the Quebec City organizer, Johnny: quiet hosting of small parties in private homes, combined with occasional group visits to American clubs such as Fernglades in Massachusetts.[1]

The first Quebec club associated with the CSA was the Heleos Health Resort, led by Adrien Decelles of St Hubert. A longtime naturist, Decelles had tried for ten years to start a group in Montreal but found that every time he mentioned organization his contacts disappeared. In 1947 Decelles and his wife, Germaine, visited the Sun Air camp in Ontario, made a good impression on the nudists there, and came away determined to act. Once home, they set up the Heleos Health Resort, with the encouragement of another sympathizer who offered land for club use, but died a year later.[2]

Through correspondence with Ray Connett, Decelles gathered about a dozen members who met in his home on Saturday evenings for cards, games, and sing-alongs. In summers the Heleos group had use of a small camp north of Montreal owned by Decelles' brother—

"the most beautiful place in the Laurentian woods." The site included a two-story log cabin that could accommodate twenty people, but the site lacked seclusion, and this caused problems later.[3]

During its first months the Heleos club operated on a cooperative basis, with members assuming organizational responsibilities. In the summer of 1948 the secretary and his family went to camp for a week and made nuisances of themselves by demanding favors such as extra meals and local transportation, so Decelles gave them a bill for the extra expenses and the secretary quit, taking with him several other members.[4]

A dozen or more couples continued to join in weekly soirées in St Hubert and attended a festive Christmas eve party at camp. But even though Decelles was "a fine friendly fellow with hospitality unexcelled," he was not aggressive in organizing or managing the club, especially after the emergence of the rival Quetans group. In 1950 a police raid at his home during a Saturday party intimidated him and the other members into closing the Heleos club.[5]

The disgruntled members of Heleos who left in August of 1948 formed a new club, which they christened Quetanners—soon shortened to Quetans. In September they held their first social gathering in the home of John and Edith for movies and refreshments. "We are just a fine, friendly group of people with the same interest in good living, sunshine, and health." A little later, the club acquired a sun-lamp for winter tanning. The Quetans were listed in both Canadian and American magazines, and formally applied to the CSA in December. But dissatisfaction with the leaders emerged among the new members. They criticized John, the former Heleos secretary, for vulgar remarks to the women at club meetings and for talking loudly and indiscriminately about nudism, the club, and club members at his restaurant. As for Paul, members and prospective members alike had a visceral aversion to him. Almost everyone breathed a sigh of relief when he ran off with another member's girlfriend.[6]

These misgivings prompted members to propose elections for a board of officers, a conditions for CSA affiliation. Shortly after the election on 5 December 1948, the founders dropped out, with John and Edith moving to Greene, Maine, where they started the Pineacres Club and claimed that "we have a wonderful under-standing among us and everything goes very smoothly." Neither the CSA nor the ASA was convinced of this. Paul resurfaced a few years later as eastern Canadian director of the International Society of Natural Living, a picture trading group.[7]

Gaetan Couture, a university engineering student who had served with the Canadian army during the war, became the new president of the Quetans. He had met other future members of the club during the summer season at the Sun Air camp and joined the Quetans in September 1948. The secretary, George Fletcher, report-ed to Ray Connett that Couture "is well liked by every member of the group. He is bilingual, tactful, a man of many interests. . . . Guy . . . is keenly interested in naturism and is willing to do prac-tically anything to help further the cause."[8]

After granting the Quetans their charter, the CSA suggested that the club explore a merger with Heleos, since the Quetans had people and Heleos had land. In May 1949 Decelles invited Quetans members to visit his camp. Couture was not impressed. Adrien had neglected to inform his brother about the visit, so Bill had invited several of his friends for the same day, leading to a suc-cession of incidents: "two men rang the bell, jumped the gate, and came running to the house; you can imagine the stampede upstairs this time (there were seventeen of us), and some just barely—yes, barely!—made it in time." Decelles came to feel that Couture wanted to "put me out of his way because of jealousy of me get-ting a big advance on him." He argued that Montreal was not big enough to support two clubs and that he had first claim because "it is not only six months that I am trying to find out but 12 years." A year later, the police raided Heleos during a meeting and took the names of everyone present. They agreed not to lay charges in exchange for Decelles' promise to disband the club, leaving the Quetans as Quebec's only recognized club.[9]

At this same time—spring of 1949—Johnny, the Quebec City

organizer, wrote to both of the Montreal clubs to establish contact and wish them well. Each responded politely but, as he complained to Connett, while Decelles invited him to visit, Couture insisted that Johnny join the Quetans first. Couture pointedly informed the CSA that the Quetans would no longer "give Johnny any opportunity of freely shopping around the various groups for likely prospects to bring into his own little private clique."[10]

Connett shared this assessment of Johnny. "He has given me repeated cause to suspect that he has a very strong 'snob' attitude. He has also snubbed the man who first undertook to organize Quebec City, and on whose land he had often sunbathed. His reasons boiled down to the fact that the man was a lower class than Johnny." Although Connett held this opinion until at least 1960, Johnny remained in place as Quebec City organizer.[11]

During 1949 the chief concern of the Quetans was locating and purchasing a campground. Couture undertook to scout out prospective lots, and in September the club arranged purchase of 70 acres of partly wooded land in the Laurentian foothills, near the village of Mille Isles, northeast of Lachute and northwest of St Jerome. But the price ($1,000) was beyond the reach of any individual member, so the club decided on a shareholding arrangement, which precipitated yet another crisis.[12]

In August, the Quetans shareholders authorized Couture to buy land in his own name on behalf of the club, since few other members were willing to be listed on record with a nudist club. The next month Couture closed the deal, and the club had its campsite. Then Couture set up a finance committee to arrange the transfer of title to the club. When a new member proposed that, since club members were apprehensive about being identified with a nudist club on a legal document, they should create a separate company, Mille Isle Development, to hold title to the land and rent it at a nominal fee to the club, Couture became apprehensive. He saw control over the land slipping through his fingers. He noted that this proposal specified that no club officers (for example, Couture) could be on the new company board, that no known nudists (again Couture) could be on the board, and that there should be no written contract between the company and the club.[13]

Couture hurriedly drafted an alternate plan, whereby he and Frank, the new president, became exclusive owners of the camp-site and the shareholders became creditors, whose investments became loans that the owners would repay. Once the shareholders approved this arrangement, Frank withdrew from ownership ("it may be that he found out that he was used by G. as a decoy"). Couture later claimed that there had never been any legal share-holders, because the receipts that he issued to contributors merely acknowledged "donations" given to purchase land; consequently "I could probably and very easily swindle all these people out of their money." But in fact Couture had called for members to buy shares in order to "raise the required capital"—a common defini-tion of a shareholder. Of course, he also noted that "the fewer the number of shareholders, the easier it would be to manage our property." When the CSA questioned his actions, Couture retort-ed that "in the event that our group should fall apart, who else but me could be better entitled to retain that property?" This shell game left Couture sole owner of the camp and sole operator of the club, one step closer to his suspected "ambition to run the nudist movement of Quebec as a private enterprise."[14]

In a circular letter to club members in December 1949, Couture announced the "wishes of a majority of the shareholders" to make the club and campground proprietary. He pledged himself to "endeavor to please all those who prove themselves to be genuine, honest, and peace-loving naturists" and expressed the hope that "the Quetans will become universally known as one of the most congenial and successful groups in existence." The way to accom-plish these objectives, as he confided to Ray Connett, was "to drop a few members who are trouble-makers." The first trouble makers were physically expelled from a meeting by Couture himself. These expulsions in turn persuaded others to leave.[15]

When the CSA president, convinced that "there is something doing in Montreal now, with a vengeance," wrote to Couture in an attempt to learn how he had gained sole control of the club, Couture replied with a massive sixteen-page typed document presenting "my version in the case of 'S vs Couture'." He also demanded that the CSA put up or shut up: "I will not resume normal activities until you give me the GO AHEAD signal." The CSA meekly gave in to Couture this time, crediting internal quarrels within the club to differences of "opinion" rather than of "fact," and offered Couture the 1950 national convention as a lure to keep his club affiliated. Now it was Couture's turn to impose conditions. "If you wish the Quetans to collaborate closely with the CSA, then the CSA must collaborate closely with the Quetans."[16]

Membership turnover became a hallmark of the Quetans. "Members are coming in and going out as fast as they come in," wrote one disillusioned Quebecer. The first time club dues were raised, nineteen of twenty-four members quit. When the shareholder dispute arose and Couture stated candidly that four more members would be thrown out if he won, the CSA president could only chuckle, "What a system!" Although the Quetans rarely had more than forty or fifty members at any one time, turnover was so frequent that hundreds of Quebecers passed through its ranks during its short history.[17]

The chief factor behind this turbulence was undoubtedly the personality of the club leader. "Unfortunately, Gaetan Couture hasn't turned out to be the man many of us thought he was." Couture had many positive attributes. He was bilingual, well-educated, a good speaker, a prolific writer, and dedicated to the spread of nudism. But he also seemed to members to be domineering, stubborn, and suspicious to the point of paranoia; "he has a one-way mind and will not take advice from any other members." As a result, Quetans became a one-man operation, a development that Couture explained as the result of a "lack of cooperation," and "no one else being willing or able to do these jobs." Yet while boasting of his myriad responsibilities—many of them blatantly exaggerated or redundant—Couture was also concerned about the impression that this self-portrayal might have on CSA officials, and hoped that they would not "construe that I am acting like a dictator and trying to run the whole show all by myself."[18]

Couture's ability to rationalize everything that he did extended to the way he ran club affairs. As he admitted to the CSA, "whether or not an official vote is taken on any matter, the decision will always be in accordance with the wishes of the majority of our members." Couture ascertained these wishes through phone calls, correspondence, private conversations, and small group discussions, always excluding the parties affected. Once he knew what he wanted the club decision to be, "there was no point in calling for a vote the result of which was a foregone conclusion." Naturally, other members disapproved of this technique: "either our conception of right is wrong or Gaetan is crazy." Such criticism only angered Couture—"I sometimes become very impatient and do even get quite mad when things don't work out the way they should"—and it was at these times that he became unpredictable or even dangerous, resulting in verbal abuse, physical manhandling, or threats of blackmail. Such threats were not taken lightly in view of the CSA suspicion that Couture had provoked the police raid that shut down the Heleos club. No wonder that members complained that "most of us are afraid to stand up to Gaetan for what we believe is right."[19]

Self-importance and self-righteousness justified much in Couture's eyes. His takeover of the club property at a time when he had invested nothing was, for him, merely a fair return for the savings that he had lived off—and the wages that he had forfeited—by not looking for work so that he would have the time to manage his takeover. "The way I figure it, my 'share' in the Quetans campsite cost me $200 of personal savings, plus about $900 in wages, or more than the total price of the land!" In fact, Couture's lack of gainful employment was a constant source complaint among Quetans members, who reported that he was always at home (although Blanche worked seasonally as a dressmaker): "He is too lazy to do any manual work, jobs have been offered to him but he always found a way to get out of accepting." Even Decelles got in a dig at his rival when he noted, "I have to support my wife, my wife don't support me."[20]

In 1949 a personal gaffe (taking unauthorized pictures) by Couture at the Sun Air club removed him from contention as officer material. But a mail ballot elected him as Eastern Director of the CSA, and Couture gushed with appreciation. "As far as the Quetans are concerned, we have received very considerable assistance from CSA; we could not even have made a start without CSA, and we could not have kept going and growing without its help." He even found kind words to say about *Sunny Trails* magazine, soon to become his *bête noire*: "when the Quetans joined the CSA family, even though ST was just a mimeographed publication, it was still our favorite, and we eagerly awaited each new issue." He even argued that the CSA should increase its dues so that it could provide more services, including a legal defense fund "which we may need very badly one of these days."[21]

In one short but eventful year Couture had silenced or expelled his critics within the Quetans and had eliminated, contained, or neutralized all other competitors in Quebec. Once the dust settled, the Quetans were able to enjoy a period of normal club activity. At the end of 1949, Couture reported 42 members, with 20 children (seldom seen and never heard at Quetans meetings, partly for security reasons). The club advertised in Canadian and American magazines; Couture acted as Canadian correspondent for *Vivre d'Abord*.[22]

Quetanners came from Montreal and nearby cities and towns. During winter members met in each other's homes in small groups. Soirées featured story-telling, songs and carols, card games (including strip poker to "break the ice"), balloon volleyball, and indoor tanning with sunlamps. In summer members worked on developing their "two million square feet of ideal playground." By the end of 1950 Couture reported the mortgage fully paid. The club intended to start work on cabins the following year.[23]

On Sunday, 29 July 1951, some club members were out at camp clearing the central field when they heard rustling in the bushes. As the women dashed into the tents to dress, Couture challenged the interlopers to reveal themselves, and "nine stalwart Provincial Police arose from the bushes, and bravely advanced upon the lone man who remained to face them." One of the police photographers entered the tent "merrily snapping many pictures," and when Couture knocked the camera away other policemen grabbed him and beat him "in the best Gestapo style." They charged Couture with "promenading in the nude on his property in public view," and his wife Blanche and another couple, the Wilsons, with "being found on property other than their own, in a state of nudity and in public view." The police had an unusual definition of "public view": "we had to crawl for more than 100 yards through the bush to get close to them without being seen." Detective-Lieutenant Trottier of the QPP Morality Squad claimed that his force had been investigating complaints of nudity for more than a year, but had lacked proof until now. He smugly added, "for a change, we didn't have to search them for evidence."[24]

It is possible that club action may have precipitated the police raid. Throughout 1950, club members negotiated with a retiree who owned a house adjacent to their camp in an attempt to acquire a ready-made clubhouse. Couture became exasperated by her inability to "make up her mind about what she intends to do with her house," and, if he treated her the way he treated club members, she may well have called in the police. Couture himself and the ASA preferred to credit Premier Duplessis, Quebec's "Little Caesar," for a politically motivated display of "morality." The editors of *Sunshine & Health* noted Duplessis' prior attacks on Jehovah's Witnesses and argued that "his party is also going to pieces" like his bridge at Trois-Rivières, and "like a drowning man Duplessis is trying to crawl up again toward popular approval by attacking and harassing a minority."[25]

The Criminal Code provision regarding nudity requires a warrant issued by the attorney general of the province before charges can be laid, but the QPP acted solely on the basis of a letter instructing them to investigate the camp for possible nudity. This outrage to civil liberty, as much as the challenge to nudism, evoked the scorn of Ray Connett in the pages of *Sunbathing for Health*.

By the time you read this the first legal test of nudism
in Canada should be ended. Its outcome, whatever it

> may be, will not be truly significant to the future of
> nudism, for it will have taken place in that never-
> never land of Canada, where progress began and
> ended approximately 1763—Quebec.[26]

As soon as they heard of the raid, club members scrounged desperately to raise the $600 bail to release Couture from jail, while the CSA and the ASA both pledged their support against this "infamous raid." The CSA executive board voted to use the CSA's general funds to help pay retainer fees for lawyers. Couture wrote shortly after his release to express his gratitude. "I don't know what else I can say to you except to thank you again for your help." At the CSA annual convention in August Ray Connett proposed that the gathering endorse the board's decisions, take up a collection, and authorize a fund-raising. Connett further proposed that the entire Publicity Fund be transferred to the Defense Fund. Later that month the board agreed to disburse funds for "any legitimate purpose connected with the Quetans case," such as fines, bonds, and legal deposits, in addition to lawyers' fees. A special Defense Committee was formed, consisting of Ray Connett in Vancouver, Bob at Norhaven, and Sam in Dorval (also a member of Norhaven). The board authorized the committee to set up a Defense Fund account at a bank in Montreal, with Sam and Margaret, a Quetans member, as co-signers. Couture reported to his members and sympathizers in October that "we are receiving full benefit" from the CSA Fund.[27] Meanwhile, Couture enlisted his own lawyer to fight the charges against him. (In addition to the camp-related charge, Couture personally was accused of distributing obscene photographs.)

The trial began in November, 1951, with reference to "strange practices which may be acceptable in other countries," but the judge noted that "this is a Catholic province, and here we observe certain beliefs and adhere to certain practices." These practices included lengthy testimony by prosecution witnesses and none by the defense, not even by Couture himself, who reported that "through flagrant distortion and misrepresentation of both the intent and the letter of the law, Judge Oscar Gagnon yesterday contrived to find me guilty." Gagnon tried to square the circle by claiming that the Criminal Code permitted nudity only among family members and invited friends but that any group of unrelated persons constituted a "public" and therefore each member of a nudist club was exposing himself or herself to the "public." Gagnon did not attempt to explain how his ruling would affect school locker rooms or YMCA swimming pools, but he did sentence Couture to six months in jail.[28]

Couture's lawyers appealed this ruling immediately, but faced several delays before a date was set. Couture speculated on the reasons for the delay: "it seems as though the judge was having a hard time making up his mind in such a way as to please his political and religious bosses, and still render a decision according to law." On 23 June 1952, Mr Justice Montpetit dismissed the charge and overturned the lower court's ruling, primarily because of the Criminal Code's stipulation requiring prior authorization from the attorney general before the laying of charges.[29]

The half-hearted tolerance that Couture and the CSA had for each other proved too fragile to withstand the tensions and emotions of the legal battle. A major bone of contention was the payment of personal expenses. When the crisis broke in August 1951 the CSA agreed to pay for "any legitimate purpose connected with the Quetans case." Its generosity was quickly put to the test as Couture flooded the board with utility bills, rent requests, and other household expenses unrelated to the trial. By November, Couture was chafing under the CSA's restrictions: tightening the purse strings and demanding details on personal expenses.[30]

At the heart of the matter was CSA inability to understand "*why* the preparation of your case has taken up your *whole* time;" why Couture made no "determined effort to get some work;" why, in short, "you don't get yourself a job?" Couture and his sympathizers tried to explain that a criminal record and the need to be free to attend court in St. Jerome at irregular times precluded steady work; he could not even get a taxi license. Couture's method of accounting also left something to be desired, in the eyes of the CSA. When *Sunny Trails* printed an expense report from Couture showing "$20.00 for taxi, etc.," Couture disputed the figures: "the undeniable truth is: *$4.00 of taxi and $16.00 of etc.*"[31]

The real issue for the CSA was that "we simply do not trust him." Couture, of course, was well aware of these suspicions. By February 1952 he went on the offensive, denouncing the "strange policies and selfish behavior" of the CSA in "grabbing for itself funds meant for the Quetans," and cutting his ties with the organization and its magazine.

> Are you now ready to abandon your unreasonable attitude and return the money where it belongs, or— must I stir up still more mud and slap you a couple more times before some sense can be knocked into your silly heads?[32]

Shortly after this blast, the Post Office informed Connett that mailing privileges for *Sunny Trails* were suspended because of its pictures, and hinted that the action was the result of complaints from "enemies in the movement in Quebec."[33]

A month later Couture issued another circular denouncing the "regrettable attitude, OUTRIGHT LIES, and ingeniously slanted interpretations issued by the CSA." He claimed to be "AT THE VERY END OF MY ROPE; UNLESS I AM RESCUED VERY SOON I MUST, THROUGH SHEER EXHAUSTION, LET GO." Couture was indeed quite despondent at this time, and confided to his few loyal supporters that he would not fight on if his pending appeal was unsuccessful. He blamed the CSA for "unrightfully holding and depriving us of more than $1000.00"; by not supporting him fully the CSA risked "scuttling the ship and imperilling us ALL." He urged supporters to contact the CSA and demand that defense fund contributions be sent "to the front line where they can be put to good and effective use."[34]

The next month Couture branded the CSA "a premature dream which cannot possibly at this present time serve the best interests of nudism in Canada," and which is "run by a small clique of over-conservative and short-sighted people in and around Vancouver." He complained that while Eastern Director he had been consulted only rarely and when he submitted proposals for discussion he had been censored. "I say again what I have repeatedly said in the past: Canadian nudism is not yet strong enough to stand on its own feet." Couture proposed dividing the CSA into three regional associations, each to become affiliated with the American Sunbathing Association, and all to be loosely coordinated in a Canadian Sunbathing Conference (a vision soon to become a reality as other easterners came to share Couture's feelings about the CSA). And although he had "no wish to 'run' such a Canadian Sunbathing Conference of the American Sunbathing Association," none the less "being the one to make the suggestion, unavoidably I would for a while be the information center for such a proposed Canadian Sunbathing Conference of the ASA." The CSA was not amused: "he must be one of those few French Canadians who are French thinking, and belittle everything Canadian."[36]

In July, Couture demanded that the CSA release its funds to him so that he could pay the lawyers, but the association preferred to deal with the lawyers directly, and this launched Couture on another tirade.

> IF YOU PURPOSELY IGNORE ME, GO OVER MY HEAD, AND NEGLECT TO INFORM ME OF YOUR DEALINGS WITH OUR LAWYERS OR ANYONE ELSE, *THEN IT IS YOUR OWN FAULT* IF I ISSUE COMMUNICATIONS THAT ARE NOT EXACTLY ACCORDING TO FACTS. . . . So now, *ACT like reliable big shots*, keep your promises, pay up![37]

When the CSA did settle with the lawyers, they also informed them that "Mr. Couture denied us any right to appeal for any further money for him, but as Mr. Couture . . . mentioned that he had received between five and six hundred dollars recently sent in for his defense, we think that you will have no trouble in collecting any balance from Mr. Couture himself."

And Ray Connett wrote personally to the lawyer to explain the procedural delays in Vancouver and to advise him that Couture had threatened legal action against the CSA. "We can only say that if the fool wishes more time in court we hope you will see that he has the money to pay for it." For its part the ASA, after watching Couture collect "18,000 dollars with no accounting but his own figures," devised a new legal aid policy to screen candidates in order to avoid subsidizing another "rebel against society."[38]

Who actually "won" in these trials was a moot point. Couture claimed a moral victory, while Quebec authorities believed they had won a victory for morality. Marcus Meed of the CSA reported on a meeting with Pacifique Plante, director of the Montreal police, later in 1955.

> He said that if the police did not know about it they could not interfere, but he would advise me not to start any nudist club in Montreal. He did not offer to shake hands at all, and I am quite sure he considered me a moral leper.[39]

Ray Connett regarded the whole experience as "a black page in our history" because thousands of dollars in legal fees bought only acquittal on technicalities rather than a decisive vindication of nudism. He felt that Couture had brought much of this trouble on himself by operating too openly, even brazenly, by not screening applicants carefully, and above all by his obsession with photographs. Couture had already got into trouble with another club by taking unauthorized pictures and resisting demands to surrender them. Yet Couture himself was well aware of the risks involved, for he cautioned another nudist about exchanging nude photos in the mail. "My only advice to him was to stop exchanging pictures and magazines, and I warned him of the severe penalties if he got caught red-handed or convicted through evidence."[40]

Couture soon ran afoul of the courts once again over nude photos, this time in Ottawa where he had moved after his trials in

Montreal. A police raid in Australia turned up pictures and addresses from around the world, including Canada, and authorities were notified. On 25 October 1957, Ottawa police raided Couture's home, seized photographs, correspondence, and personal records, and placed Couture under arrest.[41]

Couture decided to base his defense on his own Montreal precedent. Despite his vitriolic campaign against the CSA at the time of the Quetans trial, he brazenly issued an appeal to his "Very Dear Friends" asking for their support to "establish once and for all that, in Canada at least, nudists CAN lawfully send or exchange nudist photos." He assured potential contributors that "I now know how to keep costs down to a strict minimum," and—to help economize on the cost of mailing solicitations, he asked contributors to "please KEEP ON sending us additional loans UNTIL you get word from us that the battle is finally all over." But as one ASA reppresentative commented regarding Couture's "very dear friends, "they are now most reluctant to take another ride on the merry-go-round." Morality triumphed over bravado, and Couture was convicted and sentenced to six months in prison. This time there was no appeal.[42]

While Gaetan Couture had been waging his fight in four courts, Quetans members fled the club and, in many cases, nudism—at least until safe havens were established outside Quebec. This, of course, was the enduring legacy of the Quetans trial. Couture himself had written in 1949 that "if a nudist scandal occurred in the province of Quebec, it would probably set back the nudist movement in the province by about 10 years, and perhaps more." At the height of his quarrel with the CSA Couture exulted in his "victory" by asking the CSA, *WHY DON'T YOU TRY TO FORM A NEW CSA-SPONSORED GROUP IN MONTREAL? GO AHEAD AND TRY IT.*[43]

Two private clubs did operate secretly in Quebec during the mid-1950s, one an informal group of a dozen people who would gather on a small island and "have a great time in nature's sunshine," the other a more organized but unaffiliated club north of

Joliette. Unfortunately, the Quetans affair deterred many other Quebecers from starting nudism.

> I am working for the Hydro-Quebec, a government job, my boss is Premier Duplessis, and you know what he did with G. Couture. I know there is no law against our way of living, but if I ever go to court, even win my case, I would lose my job for sure.[44]

The future seemed bleak for nudism in Quebec. When a German immigrant wrote to Ray Connett about starting a new club in Montreal he received a cautionary response. "You have come to a poor part of Canada to observe the personal freedoms which we boast of to the rest of the world. . . . Perhaps you will end up moving to some other part of Canada." Ironically, when this group leader, Max Wertheim, did establish a club "in some other part of Canada," he tracked down Gaetan Couture in 1971 to learn more about the case. Couture's reply showed that he was still up to his old tricks.

> Yes, I am THE Mr. Couture you have in mind.
>
> I am now retired, expect to come into a fairly large sum in the near future, intend to buy a mobile home with part of the money, and spend the rest of my life travelling and staying at various nudist clubs all over North America.
>
> Of course, I must first of all join one club, and one or more associations. . . .
>
> We would be glad to meet you and discuss the situation in general, and possible membership in your club in particular.[45]

Presumably some of Wertheim's members in his club, East Haven, told him enough about Couture so that nothing came of this initiative.

CHAPTER EIGHT

Québec Libre

After years of stifling conservatism, on 22 June 1960 Quebecers launched the Quiet Revolution to bring Quebec's institutions and values into harmony with the modern social and economic order that had been developing in Quebec. Quebec was urban, industrial, and commercial; Quebecers were exposed to and involved with the rest of the world through trade, travel, the media, and postwar immigration. The Quiet Revolution internalized this material and attitudinal transformation.[1]

Nudists were among the first to celebrate the new atmosphere. "As far as our beautiful Province is concerned, we have had a change of government last Summer, and everybody is now feeling more free to act and talk." None the less, this was a quiet revolution: few barricades were mounted, few fortresses stormed, few pillars overthrown. Although Duplessis was gone, no one seemed eager to step into Gaetan Couture's shoes.[2]

Meanwhile, during the 1950s the first signs of more liberal behavior among Quebec nudists was the rapid growth of clubs across the borders, in Vermont and Ontario. One of the first Quebecers to attempt social nudism, even before Heleos and the Quetans, was George Fletcher of Joliette. For two summers George and some friends made the trek to North Bay. There he met Gaetan Couture, and eventually joined the Quetans club. After the raid Fletcher, who was not arrested, started looking for land outside Quebec. He spent most of his spare time scouring Ontario and Vermont, trying at first to find an island in Lake Champlain. But after visiting the Cedar Waters camp in New Hampshire in the summer of 1955, he and his associates felt that "a privately owned lake, completely surrounded by dense forest, seems to be the ideal." With the help of a "very sympathetic real estate man" George soon earmarked Long Pond, near Milton, Vermont, as the best place to begin.[3]

For a while after the end of the Quetans the group used the name Montreal Recreation Club. But in 1955 they decided "we'd rather not be associated with Montreal or Quebec," and changed the name to Forest City Lodge. Three criteria were set for membership: a current membership in the American Sunbathing Association, a substantial deposit for club fees (perhaps $100), and a congenial personality. The dozen or so prospects associated with George around 1955 were willing to accept these terms in exchange for a club with a private lake and "a nod from the law."[4]

This cautious approach did not sit well with all members of the Canadian Sunbathing Association, some of whom felt that Fletcher was "incapable" because "he keeps changing plans from day to day." But Ray Connett argued that the Montreal area could easily accommodate two clubs, one English or bilingual and one French (the East Haven club was forming at the same time). And given Fletcher's standards of admission, the clubs would have an apparent class distinction as well, with the more affluent Quebecers escaping to Vermont while the others would be left to fend for themselves—at least until East Haven found its own camp in Ontario. Connett appreciated "the care and attention you are giving to all your old contacts," even though "it is a pity that you cannot show more concrete evidence of progress in return for this investment of time and money."[5]

Fletcher's caution paid off. In 1956 his group leased ten acres on Long Pond from a local farmer, Walter Pecor. Two years later he obtained title to 35 acres on the western side of the lake and began relocating the camp there because of its larger area, more level ground, and easier access to power lines. The existence of the club became known through a feature article in June 1956 and created a local commotion, as townspeople scrambled to decide whether they should be for, against, or indifferent to the nudist colony in their midst.[6]

On Saturday, 7 June 1958, the Milton board of selectmen discussed the issue and confessed that "there is nothing we can do about it legally." In time-honored political fashion the board referred the matter to higher authorities, in this case the state attorney, Allan Bruce, who ruled that the nudist club was legal "as long as they conduct themselves in a proper manner. I have checked this thing out in the law books and I can find no law that prohibits operation of a nudist colony in Vermont."[7]

Under ordinary circumstances this ruling would have settled the question, but small-town opinion intervened and created a political ruckus that was not finally resolved until five years later. Friends of Elmer Bullock, who owned some land that touched on one corner of Long Pond, teased him about "picnicking with nudists." Bullock brooded over this razzing and finally decided to act. He contacted the local representative to the state assembly, Grace Chandler, and persuaded her to introduce a bill banning nudist clubs. He warned Fletcher that "he would do everything he could to get us put out."[8]

The guiding spirit behind much of the vocal opposition to Forest City Lodge was Father Lamb, a local Catholic priest who was one of the people taunting Bullock. Father Lamb also visited Milton's representative, Richard Branch, and persuaded him to reverse his earlier support of Forest City by threatening a boycott of Branch's store. But at this same time attorney John Cain, who had been hired by Forest City and by the ASA, met with the Catholic bishop in Burlington, who assured him that the church was strictly neutral in this matter and authorized him to inform Branch that the Church would not condone a boycott of his store.[9]

In the legislature Chandler remained committed to her bill. Although she met with Fletcher and found him to be "a very nice person," she remained opposed to the club. "I think it's a terrible thing for men, women, and children to be running around nude like that." At one point during her crusade Chandler distributed a histrionic pamphlet, "All About Nudist Colonies," inviting citizens to "read what psychiatrists, MDs and the Bible say about nudists," and urging them to "vote like respectable people!"[10]

Chandler's bill focused on the owners and operators of any property used as a nudist camp or colony; it prescribed a fine of $5,000, which was more than the penalty for second-degree murder—a fact which demonstrated the vindictiveness of the antinudist faction and which also alienated many undecided representatives. By this time too the press was openly critical of the time and expense being wasted on bills such as this which served little practical purpose.[11]

On 24 February 1959, the house committee held a public hearing at which George Fletcher was supported by several prominent citizens and organizations, including a Baptist minister and the president of the Vermont Association of Boys' and Girls' Camps. Only three people spoke for the bill, while it was impossible to schedule all those who opposed it. The committee voted 13-2 against the bill, and the chairman advised Mrs. Chandler to withdraw it, but she insisted on a House vote. On March 6 the full House voted 122 to 103 against the bill. Because of state legislative procedures, the bill could not be reintroduced for at least two years.[12]

This victory owed a great deal to the efforts of John Cain. The CSA magazine, *Canadian Sun Air*, reported that "excellent legal aid by the ASA cost $1500 but it was considered to be the deciding factor in the battle." And the ASA expressed itself well-satisfied. "Mr John Cain did an excellent job in presenting our case and in representing the ASA, even though his church and many of his close friends were fighting bitterly for the bill."[13]

While Forest City Lodge celebrated, farmer Elmer Bullock continued to brood over the taunts of friends. Four years later State Representative Elmer Bullock introduced his own bill outlawing nudism. The house general committee met on April 24, 1963, to consider alleged photographic evidence that Bullock wished to present *in camera*. Once again the "evidence" could not outweigh the testimony presented by respected citizens or Forest City's record of seven years of operation without an incident. Faced with the near-unanimous opposition of the committee, Bullock withdrew his bill in May. Cain confidently—and correctly—reported to the ASA that "it is my opinion that there will not be any future legislative attempts to ban nudism in Vermont."[14]

Today Forest City Lodge is a well-established vacation camp. Members have easy access to the many beautiful nude beach areas throughout Vermont, including a nearby island in Lake Champlain. Community opposition is a thing of the past; Fletcher has even spoken to church groups, and the club was featured in a book published by the Chittenden County Historical Society, *Look Around Colchester and Milton, Vermont*. The volume recounted the 1959 legal battle, and reported on the surprise landing on Long Pond of a seaplane, whose passengers, "after being accepted as guests of the colony, departed later with mutual respect as a result."[15]

A splinter group from Forest City Lodge founded Maple Glen. This nucleus attracted other FCL members interested in the alternative of a cooperatively owned club. Experienced British nudists formed the core of the club, but like Forest City Maple Glen also attracted many francophone Quebecers.[16]

In the autumn of 1966 the group acquired a 300 acre farm site in northern Vermont near the village of Sheldon Springs. Initially they intended to look for a small plot of 10 or 20 acres and dismissed their real estate agent's the casual remark about an abandoned farm. But as one member was driving home to Montreal after a fruitless day inspecting listings and locations, he spotted the realtor's car ahead of him and decided to look at the farm. It turned out to be the perfect choice: 300 acres of well-secluded land, less than a mile from the highway, with a farmhouse and river, all at a price the club could afford. The farmhouse became the clubhouse, shareholding members created Maple Glen

Incorporated, and in the spring of 1967 the camp opened for its first season.[17]

The cooperative organization of Maple Glen has been both an advantage and a disadvantage. It has fostered an esprit de corps among the members, who feel that "this is our club," yet the fortunes of the club are hostage to the whims of the annually elected board. Opinion divided early on whether to expand membership or to add new facilities. Eventually, the club did erect a log cabin-style clubhouse and installed an in-ground pool in 1978, in addition to tennis and volleyball courts. In 1979 Maple Glen hosted 200 visitors for the New England Conference's annual convention. But delays in decision making, the rise of full-scale resorts inside Quebec, and the persistent desire to retain a community ambience led to a decline in membership and the loss of their ASA charter.[18]

In 1955, the year Gaetan Couture won acquittal in his second court hearing, Max Wertheim, a German fur trader, arrived in Montreal. As an experienced nudist and co-founder of the Orplid club in Frankfurt, he was eager to participate in naturism in Canada and contacted Ray Connett for advice. Connett reported on the situation in Quebec, the disruption of the Quetans, and the efforts of some Quetans members to start over in Vermont, and suggested that Montreal needed another group to serve middle and working-class francophones. Multilingual Max would be well-suited for this task.[19]

Max placed an ad in Montreal newspapers announcing a "Nudist Information Center" which produced several contacts. In September 1956 the East Haven club applied to the ASA for designated group status. New Canadian Max also dutifully informed Lester Pearson of his plans, which Pearson read "with much interest," adding that "I am always glad to have imaginative suggestions of this kind."[20]

In spring 1958 some members of the club set out to search eastern Ontario for suitable campsites. They found three abandoned farms, and the final choice produced the first rift in the club, as one couple preferred the largest and most expensive farm and broke away to buy this land and create the SilvaSun Club. The others held to more modest expectations, and one of them, Jean-Guy, bought a 70 acre site on the South Nation River near Casselman, Ontario which he made available to the club until his wife forced him to choose between her and the club.[21] By this time a Montreal millionaire had joined the group and donated a large cash gift for development. Jean-Guy offered to transfer title on the land to the club in exchange for the cash, and Max accepted the offer. Until that time Jean-Guy and another well-to-do Montreal family hosted soirees in their Montreal homes to provide social events for club members. Although they balked at nude indoor parties in the Quetans style, the club did agree to buy sunlamps (against the wishes of the secretary and treasurer, who resigned and launched an attack that reached all the way to the ECSA in Ontario, the CSA in Vancouver, and Ray Connett in California).[22]

Then the club faced external challenges. The township reeve, Mr. Brisson, personally harassed the club by positioning himself outside the camp gate and interrogating visitors about "sex in the open" and by asking the club's only neighbor if he would like to make a complaint about nudist activity. Local youths applied direct pressure in the form of repeated damage to club property. When these crude attempts failed, Brisson used his official position to block the installation of electricity and to deny building permits for the construction of cabins. In both cases Max went over his head to federal and provincial authorities. Ontario Hydro agreed to install lines after the club paid a deposit. At the same time Wertheim wrote to the Ontario Municipal Commission complaining about Reeve Brisson, and the Municipalities Association assured the club that it would receive building permits. Eventually, Brisson gave up his campaign of obstruction and informed the club's local contractor that it could have whatever it wanted.[23]

Over the years East Haven has enjoyed modest but steady growth. In 1960, after several members left to join SilvaSun, the club had about two dozen families. Camp activity centered on the South Nation River, and in 1961 the club built a dock and diving board for swimming and waterskiing. Later, a fire destroyed the riverfront campsite, and the club moved upland to its present location. After years of making do with limited facilities—a natural pond and the usual games courts—East Haven added a modern in-ground swimming pool and hot tub. Today, under new management after the death of the "old warrior," who passed away in May 1994, it provides an attractive and cozy home for its fifty member families.[24]

The first defection from East Haven occurred in 1965 when Hector Morneau, a longtime member, had a disagreement with club policy and left to form his own group, the Club Naturiste Bel Air. After a year of looking for land, he found 25 acres near Alexandria, Ontario, and opened for business in 1967. Bel Air boasted a pool, a pond, a clubhouse, a sauna, the usual outdoor sports, and the novelty of parachuting courses. Membership rose steadily to 100 families, mostly French Canadians, but declined after 1974, as other clubs opened within Quebec and as Morneau tightened camp rules in order to reduce maintenance costs and to preserve the non-commercial, family-oriented ambience. "Club Bel Air understands that more than ever people are seeking a haven of peace and tranquillity where they can practice nudism in complete quietude." People gradually drifted away, and the club stopped advertising, so that no new recruits entered. By 1988, when the club closed, only a handful of members remained.[25]

A second group that spun off from East Haven resulted in the Domaine Naturiste du Québec (DNQ). The leader of the group, André Vadeboncoeur, was dissatisfied with East Haven because of its distance from Montreal and its no-liquor policy. Though anxious to set up as close to Montreal as possible, Vadeboncoeur remained cautious about locating within Quebec. So he flew along the Ontario-Quebec border in his plane scouting for campsites. Once he spotted prospective locations, he drove back for a closer look. When he found the place he wanted he sold his plane and car to pay for the land.

In October 1968 twelve couples from East Haven joined Vadeboncoeur on his *Domaine*. He announced his venture in a press conference at the Mont Royal Hotel in Montreal. The following spring the first memberships were sold, and the club started its inaugural season with twenty member families. However, his "raiding" of East Haven did not sit well with Max Wertheim, who complained to the ASA that "the way a certain André Vadeboncoeur recruited his members for his Domaine des Naturists de Quebec never has been a fair play at all." The ASA, although sympathetic, noted that members of any club have the right to shop around, and, besides, "that's a Quebec problem and we can do nothing about it."[26]

Vadeboncoeur started out with enthusiasm and "some very advanced ideas." An access road and pond were put in, and the clubhouse was built. But gradually he seemed to lose interest, and conditions deteriorated; ducks frequented the pond. After 1971, several clubs opened within Quebec and attracted many dissatisfied DNQ members. At the end of the 1973 season Vadeboncoeur approached two members, Richard and Odette Brunet, and they agreed to take over ownership in the spring of 1974.[27]

The Brunets were charter members of DNQ. Although both worked in a nearby town, they welcomed the opportunity to change careers. Because they were well-known to other members, the change in ownership revitalized the club; many who had considered leaving now chose to stay. Richard set to work building and renovating. He expanded the clubhouse, added a bar and disco, installed an in-ground pool, expanded the children's playground, and improved the roads, to which members gave colorful names: rue des gallants, rue des sansculottes, rue des sexentriques.[28]

Since 1974 the club has grown to more than 100 member families. Although most are French Canadian, nearly half are bilingual. Members come from Montreal, Ottawa, and nearby smaller towns such as Rigaud, Hawkesbury, Sorel, and Valleyfield. The club advertises in newspapers, and the proprietors occasionally appear on radio talk shows. In 1980 the name was changed to Club Naturiste Richard Brunet because the Liquor Control Board of Ontario balked at giving a permanent license to a "Quebec" club.[29]

The CNRB developed a unique *esprit de corps.* In the spring of 1979 some members decided to organize a newsletter to announce camp events and to serve as a forum for members' creativity: letters "if anyone writes," cartoons "if anyone draws," and a special column for "spicy gossip" which never lacked material. Another example of CNRB camaraderie is a camp song written by Marcel and sung on outings, especially volleyball competitions where the club more than holds its own.

> We love the life of fresh air
> Tanning our backsides in the bare
> At DNQ volleyball
> Is everyone's first call
> Our teams are all a blast
> Because our players are so fast.[30]

At the end of the 1983 season members gave the Brunets a plaque celebrating "two golden owners who have made DNQ the ideal place to live." The following spring the Brunets hosted a dinner for the club, at which they honored the forty-five members who had joined during Vadeboncoeur's tenure. Vadeboncoeur himself returned in the 1990s.[31]

The last Quebec club to locate in Ontario, Ann-Yvon, was founded in 1977 by two other members of East Haven who sought to foster a "family atmosphere free of cliquishness." They bought 44 acres near Club Bel Air and installed a clubhouse, a pool, and sports facilities. Membership remained small, however, and eventually the club became a private retreat for the owners and friends.[32]

By 1969, despite an abortive attempt to form a nudist club inside Quebec—the Fondation de Vitalité Las Eden—it became increasingly apparent that Quebec now more than ever was ready for nudism *chez nous.* Once the Quiet Revolution intersected with the sexual revolution of the sixties Quebec exploded into liberation.[33]

The first successful club was the Paradis Terrestre, located on the beautiful 240-acre site of an old scout camp in the Laurentians. The wooded and hilly terrain, with more than 300 camp sites, featured a waterfall, lake, and river, to which had been added an indoor swimming pool and clubhouse. The club was set up in the autumn of 1971, and opened for its first season on 12 May 1972.[34]

The original owners, Paul and Marcel Lépine, were former members of DNQ. Twenty six families joined the Lépine brothers on the trek to Chertsey in order to finally have a Quebec club in Quebec. The new club was well received by the community, even though its neighbors included church camps and shrines. The mayor of St Theodore de Chertsey anticipated "a very substantial source of revenue" for the town.[35]

Paradis Terrestre quickly took on the commercial gloss typical of many American clubs and even joined the ASA in 1975 (but quit when few American tourists arrived). Publicity events such as the World Queen of Nudism contest in 1976 were well promoted—the club published its own newspaper, *Paradis Terrestre*—and helped increase membership to 350 families, or more than 1,000 individuals. In 1978 the third owner, Gérard Lépine-Fontès, reorganized the club to create a condominium-style residential community: members owned their lots and homes while the Paradis Terrestre company owned the common areas. After he sold his interest, Lépine-Fontès attempted to start a similar community adjacent to the Pommerie club south of Montreal, but this project was foiled by local authorities. Meanwhile, the proliferation of other clubs in Quebec, and the frequent changes in ownership, led to a decline in membership and the eventual closing of Paradis Terrestre. But for many years the club was truly "the school of nudism" for Quebec.[36]

The next club to open within Quebec was the Club Naturiste Laurentien, near St. Michel de Wentworth, north of Lachute. The club spread over 500 acres, embracing three lakes, woods, and mountains, and offered swimming, sailing, canoeing, hiking, and mountain climbing, in addition to volleyball, badminton, archery, and other traditional camp games. In winter the club featured cross-country skiing, tobogganing, ice skating, and hockey. Club Laurentien, owned and operated by a family from the Brownsburg area, was fully bilingual. Although the camp operated as a nudist club during 1973 and 1974, the owners decided to open the grounds to clothing-optional activities, which attracted too many voyeurs for the comfort of the nudists, who left in droves—hastened perhaps by "blackflies, horseflies and mosquitoes," which "made the situation intolerable for most." The club closed down soon afterwards, and the land became the site of an upscale four season residential development.[37]

The Domaine Naturiste Adam et Eve was founded by Elmen Tremblay in 1973, after years of waiting. Tremblay was a naturalist as well as a naturist, and from the beginning his club appealed to people who preferred naturism over nudism. The camp comprised 250 acres in the Laurentians, near the resort of Estérel, and boasted a lake, a heated in-ground pool, a sauna, a whirlpool, and a hilltop sundeck that provided a view for fifty miles. The unique commitment to nature, expressed in weekend discussions on flora and fauna conducted by a member who was also a professor of ecology, attracted 125 member families. But other policies, including a flip-flop commitment to nudity one year and clothing-optional status the next, along with Tremblay's retirement in 1978, led to a rapid decline in numbers and eventual closing.[38]

The Club de Nudistes Oasis was set up in late 1973 by André and Georgette Bélanger, former members of the Paradis Terrestre who became disenchanted with its commercialism. At the outset, Bélanger attempted to organize indoor winter meetings to keep members together during the off season. On the first night at an indoor pool in a private gym on Boulevard Métropolitain in Montreal some 100 adults were surprised by a loud noise outside. When they opened the door, several police rushed in and nearly fell into the pool. They had arrived to check on Bélanger's license for alcohol, and, after seeing that everything was in order, they left. But the experience sufficiently dampened members' enthusiasm that no more swim nights were held, and Bélanger relied instead on publicity events such as nude theater featuring the Libérés troupe from Forest City Lodge, which presented *The Dream of Jonathan* to audiences of several hundred non-nudists. Despite a change in ownership during the 1980s Oasis remains a large and very popular club, "one big happy family," with activities for members of all ages.[39]

The Royaume de l'Eden (not to be confused with a short-lived club in the Eastern Townships called L'Eden des Nudistes) was founded in 1976 by some members from Oasis who wanted more "fun." The owners invested $300,000 in the clubhouse alone, in addition to all the usual outdoor facilities. For publicity Eden presented nude theater (until a fire destroyed the clubhouse and the arsonist) and erotic fashion shows. Eden became one of Quebec's most popular and successful clubs, attracting 2,000 people on some summer weekends. In 1989 Eden was sold to a club member, who rebuilt the clubhouse. But increasing commercialization and liberalization started to drive members away in the 1990s—many of them back to Oasis (too much "fun" perhaps).[40]

The first of two clubs to locate south of Montreal was Vallée Rustique, located in the Appalachian foothills of southern Quebec. It opened on 24 June 1974 and was the first of the new clubs to affiliate with the ASA. Owner Normand Côté invested substantially in the club, which was the first in Quebec to offer tennis courts. Members could also take advantage of the four miles of nature trails winding along the wooded hillside. After fifteen years of successful operation Côté retired and new owners, Gilles and Geneviève, took over in 1991.[41]

La Pommerie was founded in 1976 by French-born Dr Jean Marcel, who came to Canada for university study and remained here, becoming employed by the government. He had early childhood experience with nudism on a family visit to Finland, and after several years in Dahomey setting up the Collège

Polytechnique Universitaire he returned to Canada by way of France, where he spent some time at naturist resorts in Corsica. Once back in Canada he joined Paradis Terrestre but, dissatisfied with the climate conditions there, he searched for a location closer to Montreal. La Pommerie boasts of being open for business while other Quebec clubs are still shovelling snow.[42]

La Pommerie is unique among Quebec clubs for its commitment to naturism; in fact, if push came to shove, Boucher said that he would opt for naturism over nudism. He has held this philosophy since at least 1975, when he responded to a survey of Quebec naturists by asserting that "the genuine nudist is an ecologist, an observer of beauty, truth, and health." This attitude became enshrined in the "Trait d'Union" issued by Pommerie to all members and applicants.[43]

The naturist emphasis at Pommerie is evident in the 1,000 apple trees and in the courses in ecology, ceramics, crafts, yoga, and other naturist topics. Not surprisingly, Pommerie has appealed to the urban professionals of Montreal: "it quickly rallied those who want something more than a suntan, tennis, and Molson's." Membership totals several hundred families, and reservations are made months in advance. In 1995 Boucher sold the club to a group of members, who continue its operation as an "ecological and naturist center."[44]

The Club Naturiste Adam et Eve in Sainte Brigitte des Saults was started in 1972 by Arthur Chartrand. On 100 acres, the club provided a pool, a pond, volleyball, badminton, horseshoes, petanque, and, in winter, cross country skiing and snowmobiling. The club held annual royalty contests, which were opened to the public in the mid-1970s and attracted hundreds of spectators. After Chartrand sold the club in the autumn of 1977 the new owners upgraded the entertainment by offering Miss Nude Quebec contests, which attracted thousands of viewers and received media coverage. These spectacles did not sit well with all members, some of whom left to form their own clubs. Although the contests ceased in the early 1980s, the experience had clearly changed the ambience of the club. In 1986 the Adam and Eve Club was advertising as a "key club for liberated people" and was featured in the tabloid *Photo Police* under the headline, "Nudist Camps are for Swingers."[45]

In 1976 a dozen members of Adam and Eve decided to form the Loisirs Air Soleil camp on 150 acres along the St Francis River between Richmond and Drummondville. "We wanted a club at once entertaining and relaxing. We wanted nudists to enjoy themselves without disturbing their neighbor who prefers peace and quiet." About ten years later, after much family oriented growth and activity, some members founded another club, Domaine Soleil de l'Amitie, near St Cyrille. The Air Soleil cooperative sold the club to a proprietary owner in 1995, after reaping a bonanza from the sale of industrial sand.[46]

The largest campground in Quebec belonged to the Domaine Naturiste Le Cyprès in Notre Dame des Anges, northwest of Quebec City. Le Cyprès was situated on 560 acres of wooded country, with a ten kilometer canoe route along the Batiscan River. Patrick Couture started the club in 1976 as Camping Notre Dame des Anges. It was the first club near Quebec City and attracted members from the provincial capital and from other regional centers. For publicity Couture staged Venus de Québec contests. Such events aroused the ire of the local curé, and suspicious villagers tore down directional signs as fast as they were put up.[47]

In 1978 Roland Dion, a restauranteur from Quebec City, bought the club and developed the facilities while continuing to emphasize the wilderness camping. In 1980, 1,500 families stayed at Cyprès, with up to 400 people present on some weekends. This investment and activity helped change local attitudes towards the club. In 1988 Dion retired and sold Cyprès to two families, who developed the club further by adding an in-ground pool, but disagreements over the scale of expansion led one family to sell out to the other. In 1994 two new member families purchased the camp, and continue to operate it as a naturist resort.[48]

In 1981 several members of Cyprès, dissatisfied with the club and the distance to Quebec City, established the Camping Nature Détente near St Raymond, less than half the distance to the capital. The grounds center around a lovely spring-fed lake with a wide sand beach. The club remained aloof from its counterparts and from the Quebec Federation of Naturism, but this reserve moderated after the opening of yet another club in the Quebec City area, L'Avantage, which took over a former youth camp and opened in 1987 with two large inground pools, a clubhouse, a restaurant, a bar, sports facilities, children's playground, and 90 acres of wooded land with a river, all less than half an hour from Quebec City. L'Avantage was operated by Pierre Fillion, a naturist since 1969, and his American wife, Marilyn, and was one of the few Quebec clubs to offer bilingual services. But competition in the Quebec city area led Fillion to convert the club to a conventional camp, Air d'Été, at the end of the 1991 season. Nature-Détente moved to take up the slack and affiliated with the FQN.[49]

In northwest Quebec Les Amis de la Nature started a camp near Val d'Or, with sauna, clubhouse, lakefront beach, and volleyball. By 1979 the club had attracted two dozen families, but slow growth prompted the it to offer clothing-optional as well as nudist activities. In 1995 a new club, Cité du Soleil, opened in the Lac St Jean area. And throughout Quebec there are small groups of friends who share cottages or woodland in an informal manner, without affiliation with other clubs and organizations.[50]

The 1970s gave Quebecers their very own Florida nudist club for those long Quebec winters. Quebec nudists traditionally frequent Cypress Cove, Lake Como, Sunny Palms, and other Florida clubs. It was only a matter of time before a club opened there, run by Quebecers for Quebecers. Ads in the tabloid *Nudistes du Québec* promised that here "our kind can meet again among friends and speak French: no problems with translation." Jean Paul Veilleux, a Quebec businessman and former member of DNQ and the Sunny Palms club, opened Jupiter Sunshine Gardens (JSG) in the mid-1970s, after a two year battle with zoning officials, prompted by the *fait accompli* of Veilleux in converting a ten acre homesite into a nudist park. JSG featured a large inground pool, a pond, and tennis, volleyball, petanque, badminton, and shuffleboard courts, as well as swings and trampolines for the children. Membership in Jupiter Sunshine Gardens was mostly Québécois, especially the on-site residents. Visitors included Americans and Canadians attracted by ads in the ASA *Bulletin* and in *Nudistes du Québec*. In December 1978 an All Florida Days celebration, with contests in volleyball, tennis, shuffleboard, and swimming drew 1,000 visitors. Continuing battles with local officials led Veilleux to sublet and then sell the club. He himself moved to another club nearby.[51]

Clubs attracted members through media reports, advertising, and word of mouth. During the 1970s and 1980s several Quebec clubs operated successful information booths at the annual Camping Show at Place Bonaventure in Montreal, and at the Family Vacation Show and the Leisure Show.[52]

In order to promote their mutual interests, six club owners met in April 1976 to discuss common concerns, including shared purchasing power, government lobbying, and membership issues. But the chief concern of the Association of Nudist Clubs of Quebec came to be the organization of inter-club volleyball competitions, which were taken very seriously indeed. The Quebec Volleyball Association provided the judging, while Molsons provided the trophies. Over the years CNRB and Air Soleil have distinguished themselves on the courts, not only in Quebec but at the Nude Volleyball Superbowl at White Thorn Lodge in Pennsylvania. Some club owners tried to address other issues such as publicity and a code of ethics. In the 1990s club owners formed yet another trade association to promote their interests without interference by the FQN.[53]

A second form of publicity for nudism was the presentation of nudist plays at various clubs for the general public. Club Laurentien offered the Broadway play *Barely Proper* in the summer of 1974, while Adam and Eve presented *If Daddy doesn't like it, he'll have to go along with mummy, my pal, the maid, and me*. But the principal theatrical troupe involved was Les Libérés, a group that originated among club members at Forest City Lodge. In 1970 Beaujean wrote a skit, *The Initiation*, which was presented at Forest City over the Labor Day weekend. During the next several years Les Libérés offered new plays at FCL, and their reputation spread. In 1974 they performed *We Nudists* at Paradis Terrestre and at the University of Montreal. The next year saw *Future Shock*, about an author in 2024 reminiscing on how his nude society, ruled by women, had changed from 1974. The group also presented skits at Paradis Terrestre during the Olympiade in 1976. In 1977 they presented *The Dream of Jonathan* to audiences of several hundred at Oasis, where they found their greatest response. Before each performance André Bélanger showed slides illustrating life at Oasis.[54]

A third publicity event was the wrestling gala hosted by both Oasis and Paradis Terrestre during the summer of 1977. On 26 June Oasis presented Edouard Carpentier against Tarzan Tyler; Gino Brito and Tiger Jackson; Raymond Rougeau versus Bull Gregory; and Little Brutus against Little Beaver. On 20 August Paradis Terrestre featured Mad Dog Gagnon, Lionel Provost, Guy Ranger, and Ski Doo Bombardier.[55]

The most conspicuous form of publicity for nudism was the bi-weekly tabloid *Nudistes du Québec,* a product of Quebec's sexual revolution that was published by Jean Marc Provost between 1976 and 1983. It offered regular reports on club activities and often featured full-page articles about individual clubs and special events, especially the Miss Nude Quebec contests, some sponsored in part by Provost. He also organized group vacations to Jupiter Sunshine Gardens in Florida. But over the years, as clubs found other ways to advertise and as the FQN set out to promote nudism in a more respectable manner, nudism came to be overshadowed by articles and photographs that were exclusively sexual and pornographic in nature. The Association of Nudist Clubs of Quebec collectively, and various club owners individually, complained vociferously about the calibre of *Nudistes du Québec,* but Provost replied that "one must above all respect the freedom of choice of everyone. You may not like part of the paper, but that doesn't necessarily make it bad."[56]

Whatever readers might think, *Nudistes du Québec* was a prominent feature in the history of nudism during the 1970s, selling tens of thousands of copies of its biweekly editions. Many club members, and many members of the FQN, first learned about Quebec nudism on its pages when it was the only nudist publication available and Provost was the only person promoting nudism. (A decade later Provost popped up as a tabloid reporter for *Photo-Police* with a sensationalist article critical of the nudism he once promoted.)[57]

The FQN sponsored alternative "clubs" or chapters called "sections," to provide naturist activities to people whose careers and family status precluded membership in clubs, and particularly to supplement the short outdoor season with indoor swimming and games. Regional chapters were set up in Montreal and in Ottawa (1978), Quebec City (1980), Mauricie (1982), the Eastern Townships (1984), Abitibi, South Shore, and Saguenay (1985), and North Shore and Richelieu (1986). Only a few of these chapters succeeded in providing alternative nudist facilities for members, but those few demonstrated the great need for such activities, particularly indoor winter swimming.

For the first few years the Montreal chapter *was* the FQN. At one time the Montreal Olympic Stadium offered the use of its pools to the FQN, but it declined because the pools were too large and too deep, and the room was too drafty. Instead, it rented a pool at the CEGEP Maisonneuve and advertised in the media in order to attract the public. Many novices tried naturism at these swims, and some joined the FQN or one of the landed clubs. In 1986 the Montreal section rented the YMCA at Pointe St Charles. The move produced an effect "like night and day," as the new location, the broader range of activities, and the more convenient time (Saturdays instead of Thursdays) gave everyone "a breath of fresh air." Attendance climbed from sixty singles to one hundred adults and twenty children per week. On special occasions such as open house nights or inter-section visits from Quebec, Shawinigan, or Sherbrooke, attendance topped two hundred. In the course of a year 2,000 to 3,000 people attended the swims, all nude except for the lifeguards, even though the FQN suggested "they would be more comfortable if they had the same costume as we in the FQN." In later years some guards did accept the FQN "costume."[58]

In 1988 the *merde* hit the *ventilateur* when the *Montreal Daily News* exposed "Nude Volleyball? The 'Y' Bares It." Reporter Grace Wong described the FQN winter activities during the past two years and quoted the director of the Pointe St Charles Y as saying "I have no problems renting out the facility to a legitimate group like the Federation." Unfortunately, the publicity proved too much for the Y and its donors, and the FQN, now at the YMCA Guy Favreau, had to pack its bags and move to the CEGEP Maisonneuve, until in 1990 it acquired the use of a private recreation complex on Laurier street which provided a swimming pool, children's pool, hot tub, volleyball, badminton, and exercise room.[59]

The Quebec City regional chapter was established in the autumn of 1979 and immediately attempted to arrange winter swims. After being rejected by the local CEGEP, it made arrangements with the YMCA and started the first season in October 1980. Like the Montreal chapter, the Quebec group advertised publicly. Twenty-seven people attended the first night, but soon nearly one hundred people came to the weekly sessions, more than two thousand during the season. Unfortunately, a change in regional leadership contributed to the decline of indoor activities in Quebec after 1989.[60]

The Ottawa-Hull-Gatineau area was represented at first by the Naturist Group of Ottawa, an autonomous organization established in 1978 which formally joined the FQN the following year. Although the population of national capital area suggested great potential for nudism, growth was slow. The Ottawa Naturist Group found little response to its efforts to organize winter activities. The situation did not improve after the group became the FQN's Ottawa Section in 1979. When the FQN advertised "indoor naturist activities" in 1985, only a dozen people showed up, prompting the area organizer to comment that "even an earthquake couldn't budge the Ottawa populace." In 1987 the University of Quebec at Hull halted negotiations out of concern that "the students will want to bathe nude also." Not until 1990 would the good citizens of Ottawa enjoy winter skinnydipping, under the auspices of a new club, the Ottawa Naturists.[61]

Federation members first tried to organize activity in the Eastern Townships in 1982 but met with little success. In 1984 they arranged to rent the YM/YWCA in Sherbrooke, but attendance was never sufficient to cover the costs of renting the pool, and the experiment soon stopped. In 1983 the Mauricie chapter rented the Cultural Center in Shawinigan and hosted five hundred people each season. And in 1986 the Saguenay chapter rented a private swimming school in Chicoutimi after a local hospital refused to accommodate the naturists because of "the type of activity which you envision."[62]

The FQN also set up various groups to help organize special interest activities. The youth group started in 1980 to structure activities and events for young singles at the landed clubs. Inter-club volleyball competitions topped the agenda, but members pursued other games and sports, arranged dances, and went on group outings to free beaches. Several of the larger clubs welcomed the youth group in exchange for occasional help such as spring cleaning. Closely related was the special "naturist adventure" chapter formed in 1987 to organize a Canadian tour by visiting European youths. The canoe-camping group organizes canoeing trips to the Mauricie, Mount Tremblant, Papineau, and Vérendrye provincial parks. The singles group organizes trips within Quebec, while the FQN travel group has journeyed to Cuba, Guadeloupe, and Mexico, among other destinations.[63]

Publicity, general interest, and curiosity all resulted in the rapid growth of nudism in Quebec during the 1970s as ten clubs attracted several thousand members. Growth continued into the 1980s, but peaked around 1985. Once nudism became socially accepted, members comparison-shopped among various leisure activities or took nudist vacations outside Quebec, in the United

States, the Caribbean, and Europe. The economy, the climate, and the retirement of many of the original club owners also limited the expansion of nudism. Today, nudism is as well represented in Quebec as in any other province, but as in the rest of Canada the participation rate lags far behind Europe.

> Naturists in the rest of Canada may well look upon their québécois counterparts with envy. There are more clubs and free beaches in "Lower Canada" than in the remaining 9 provinces combined. The degree of tolerance for nudity in most areas is unparalleled in the rest of the country, with a couple of local exceptions on the West Coast. In short, Quebec may seem to come as close to a naturist paradise as contemporary society and the Canadian climate allow.[64]

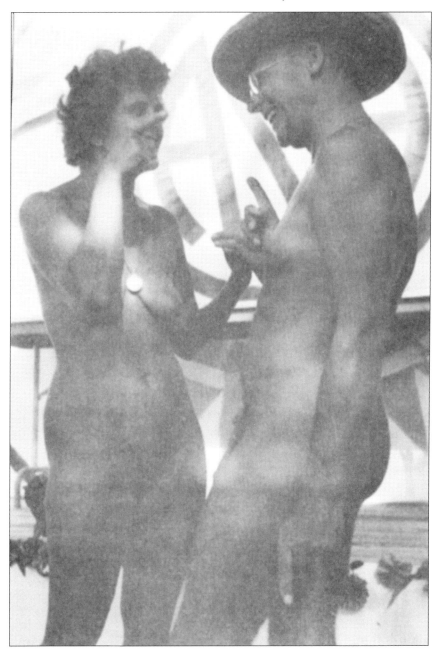

East vs West: Mary of TGS meets Ray at the ASA convention.

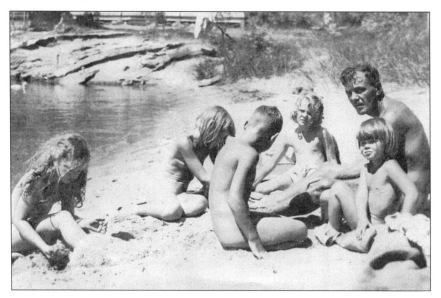

The Sun Air Freedom Lovers at Belle Isle.

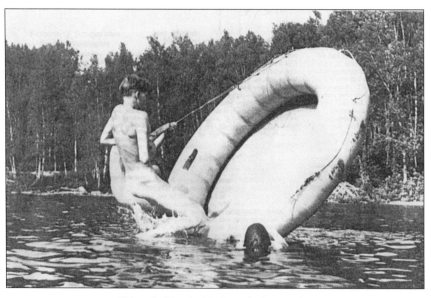

Kids splashing in Norhaven's Otter Lake.

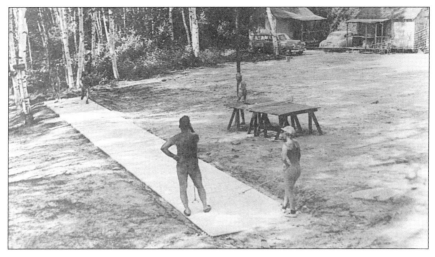

Shuffleboard at Norhaven.

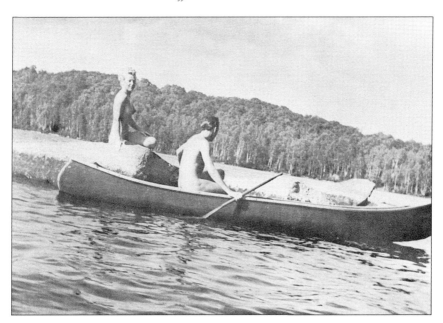

Canuding on Otter Lake at Norhaven.

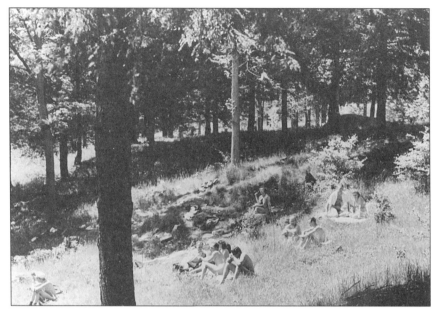

The Sunglades Club of Toronto.

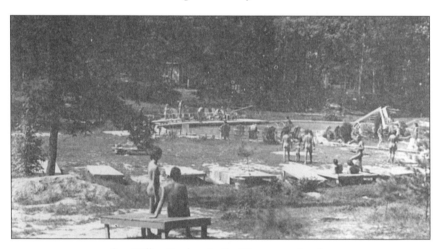

Sun Valley Gardens in the Niagara peninsula.

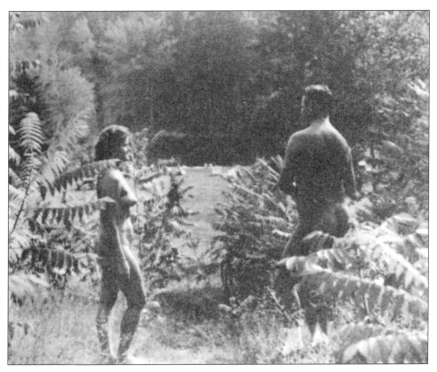

Eddy and Mary, founders of Glen Echo, start planning.

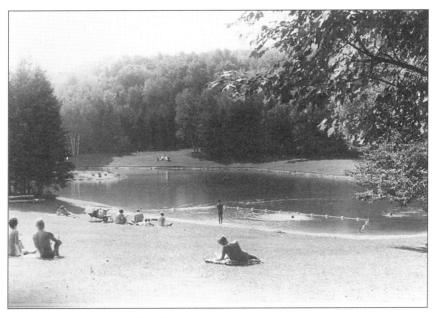

Glen Echo after years of hard work.

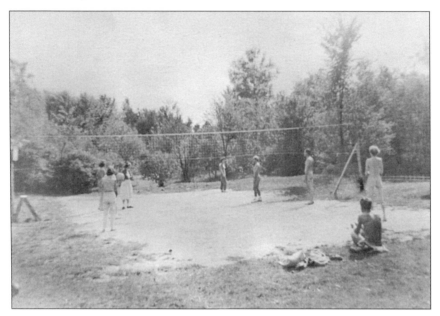

Volleyball at the London Sun Club.

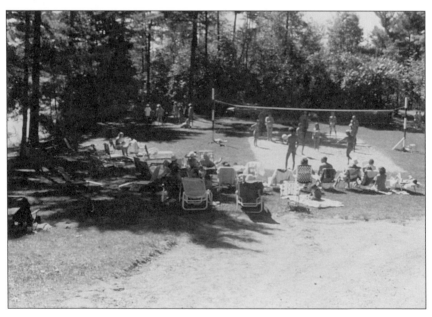

Volleyball at the Lakesun Club near Kingston.

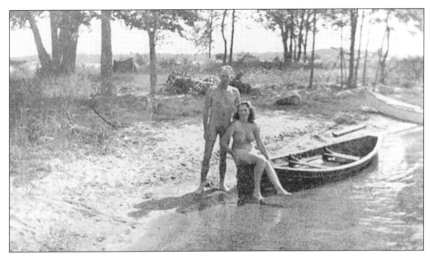

Adrien and Germaine Decelles, founders of the Heleos Club.

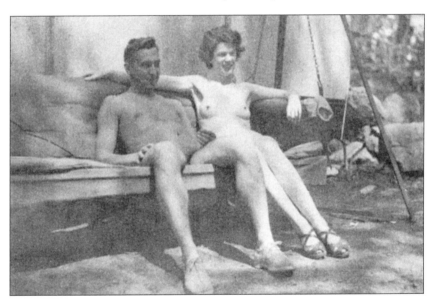

Gaétan and Blanche Couture, leaders of the Quetans Club.

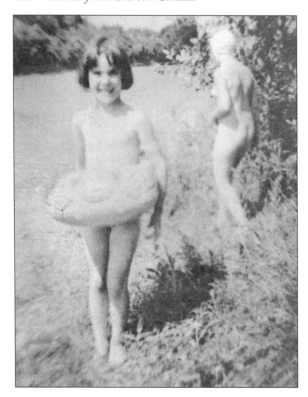

The early East Haven club on the South Nation river.

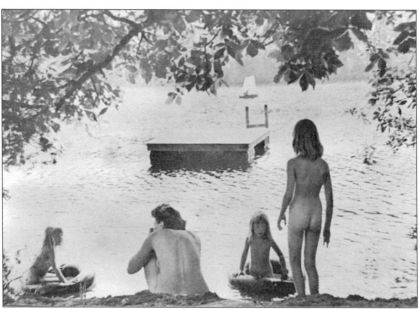

Forest City Lodge on Long Pond in Vermont.

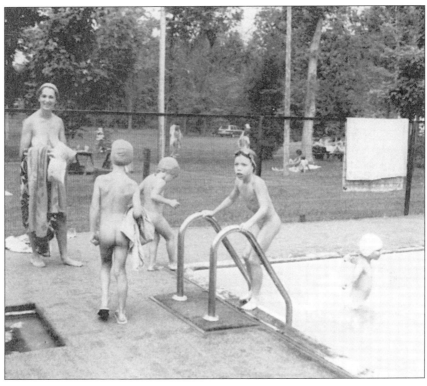

Bel Air, near Alexandria, ON.

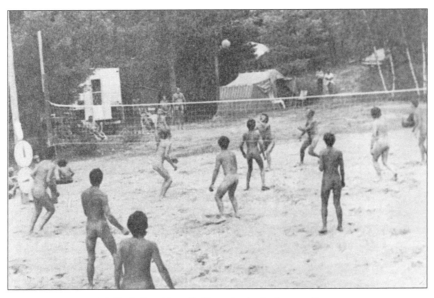

Volleyball at Paradis Terrestre in the Laurentians.

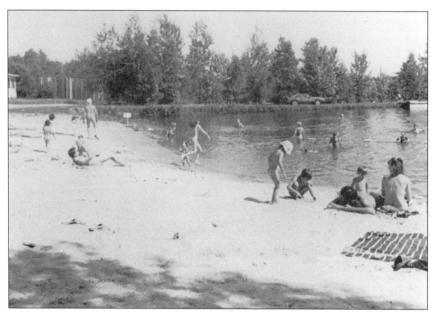

Club Oasis, north of Montreal.

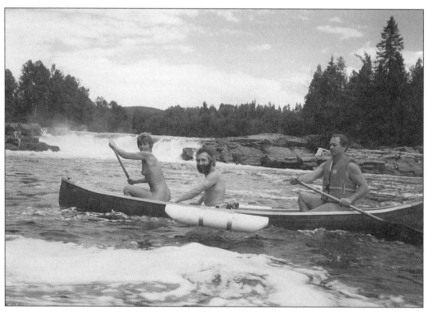

Canuding on the Batiscan River at Le Cyprés.

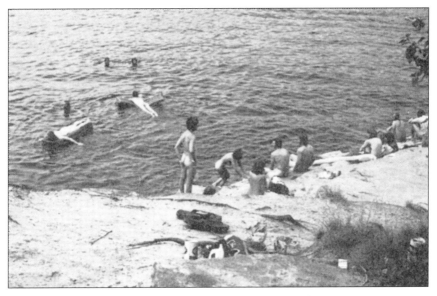

An informal nude beach near Montreal.

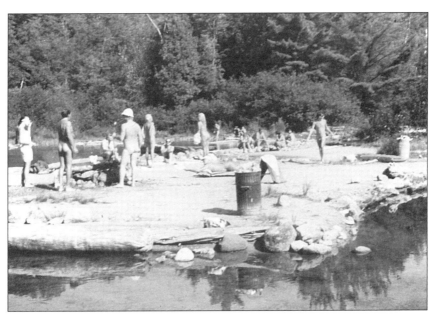

The nude beach at Meech Lake.

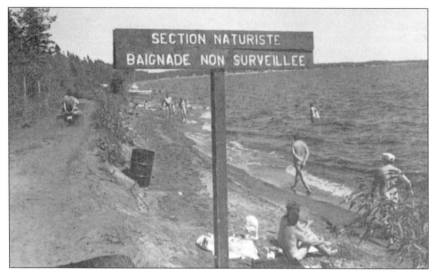

The free beach at Point Tailllon on Lac St. Jean.

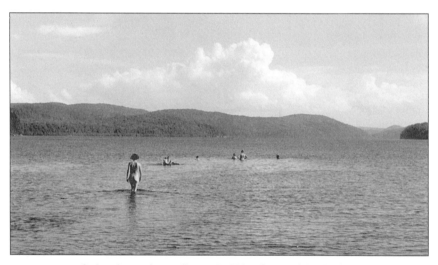

Swimming and canuding at Le Vérendrye park in Quebec.

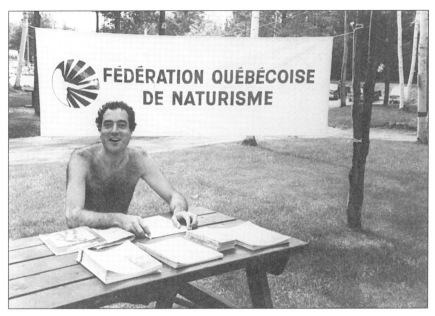

Michel Vaïs, founder and first president of the FQN.

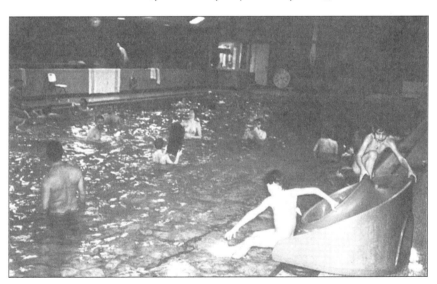

Indoor swimming sponsored by the FQN.

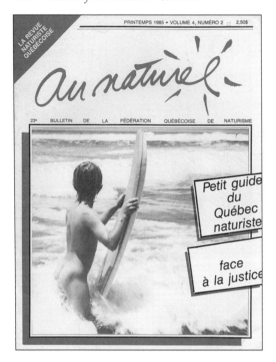

Au Naturel, *former magazine of the FQN. Superseded by* Naturisme Québec.

An early version of Going Natural, *magazine of the FCN. Wreck Beach on the cover.* Going Natural *has appeared in full-color format since 1998.*

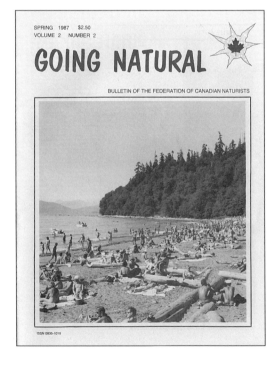

CHAPTER NINE

A Mari usque ad Mare

C anada's free beaches range from Bare Ass Beach in Saskatoon to Bare Bum Beach in Brantford and the Bare Skin Club in Selkirk; from Ear Lake in the Yukon to Lucy Lake in Nova Scotia. But the most popular free beaches in Canada are in British Columbia, home to Canada's one and only "world class" nude beach, and in Quebec. The diverse provincial experiences with free beaches demonstrate the popularity of nude recreation in Canada, the possibility of legal toleration, and the difficulty in securing permanent official recognition on the European model.[1]

British Columbia offers an ocean, inland lakes, and rivers in wooded mountainous country with Canada's mildest year-round climate. It features a variety of free beach areas, from Long Beach in the Pacific Rim National Park near Tofino to Three Mile Beach in Penticton. Virtually all major cities have their own skin beaches. In Victoria there is Island View Beach, where the only official action has been to separate the nude from the textile bathers, and Prior Lake in Thetis Lake Park west of the city, where nude sunbathing has been tolerated since the 1970s.[2]

On the mainland, just up the coast from Vancouver, lies Howe Sound, a wide open area with numerous islands, where a group of men went "sailing, drifting, climbing, lounging" (and swimming) during the 1930s. Brunswick Beach on Howe Sound gained notoriety in 1992 when, after twenty-five years of nude sunbathing at the east end of the beach, homeowners complained that nudists were "making a spectacle of themselves" and obtained an injunction barring anyone from "causing or creating a nuisance publicly by appearing, being, basking, parading, or bathing in the nude."

Nudists organized with assistance from the Wreck Beach Preservation Society, and the Brunswick Beach Bares got the injunction set aside in BC Supreme Court on the grounds that only the attorney general has authority to restrain a public nuisance.[3]

Inland, the Okanagan Valley has innumerable beach areas such as Nipple Point in Salmon Arm. And the hot springs of BC offer another unique free beach experience: Hot Springs Cove north of Tofino; the Sooke River potholes near Victoria; Meager Creek Hot Springs and Skookumchuk Hot Springs north of Vancouver on the Lillooet River; and Sheep Creek Hot Springs in the Kootenays.[4] But one beach in BC transcends all others and has become the premiere nude beach in Canada, and that is Wreck Beach in Vancouver.

The first reported nude beach in Vancouver appeared in 1936. In that depression year some unemployed young men lacking funds for conventional beachwear and locker rental decided to forego formal attire and use one of the many secluded beaches in Vancouver "in complete naturalness." The group cleared debris off a stretch of sand alongside the Siwash Rock in Stanley Park and disported themselves until "Mrs Grundy" complained and the police moved in. This evoked a public response, and one letter to the *Vancouver Sun* observed that "nowadays nudist bathing is such a common thing almost all over the world that it doesn't seem too much to ask that it be permitted in reason in Vancouver."[5]

Stanley Park continued to be the gathering place for sun-bathers for a few more years. "They gather daily in suitable weather on an isolated bit of the seashore. . . . Their presence has been known and winked at by park police for years." But one fine day in March 1947 a dedicated citizen camped in the woods for three days to observe these heinous flaunters of public morality, whom he then zealously reported to the police. The media had a field day with Mr Peeper, whom Jack Scott of the *Vancouver Sun* described as "the Moron of the Week" with his "beady eyes eager to discover evil." The park police shrugged off the incident and the publicity. "There has been nude bathing within the vicinity of this famous rock since time beyond the memory of the white man."[6]

By this time the focal point of nude sunbathing in Vancouver had shifted to Wreck Beach, where it has remained ever since. In the 1920s construction of the University of British Columbia (UBC) campus on Point Grey brought people to Wreck Beach, which lies along the base of the cliffs of the peninsula, and some of them started to take advantage of its seclusion for nude swimming and sunning.[7]

Unorganized nudity on the beach continued after the Second World War. Then came the 1960s and the counterculture movement, with its sympathy for a freer and more natural way of life. More and more people gravitated to Wreck Beach, prompted by the "Nude-In" promoted in the *Georgia Straight* underground paper. Eventually the inevitable complaints were filed, the police moved in, and arrests were made. In August 1970 thirteen people were arrested on Wreck Beach and charged with "committing an indecent act." One of those arrested, Sheila Beaupre, was fined $50, but the BC Supreme Court overturned her conviction in January 1971 on the grounds that she had been indicted under the wrong section of the Criminal Code. The Crown then dropped charges against the others arrested the same day. From that point on there has been no arrest for "being nude in a public place" on Wreck Beach itself, but one woman Mountie candidate was dropped from the force for revealing her secret identity while sunbathing nude on the beach.[8]

The Wreck Beach Defense Fund was a product of the 1960s counterculture in Vancouver. The underground paper *Georgia Straight* coordinated a "Nude-In" on the beach immediately after the arrests in August 1970. On 23 August several hundred nudists gathered on the beach to swim, sun, read, play, and listen to music. This time police were conspicuous by their absence.[9]

Throughout the 1970s the popularity of Wreck Beach increased, and thousands of nudists freely disported themselves

on warm summer days. But although the police had learned to
live with the nudity, there were others who had not, and in 1977
one of them, the pentecostal preacher and alderman Bernice
Gerard, saw a golden opportunity for righteous indignation and
free publicity. On 10 July Gerard and about 100 "citizens for
integrity" marched along Wreck Beach in a crusade against nudity. The good citizens came armed with cameras to do battle for
morality. The nudists wore fig leaves in deference to the preacher's biblical training, and carefully dressed their pet dogs.[10]

By the late 1970s and early 1980s Wreck Beach became so popular—drawing thousands of visitors every weekend—that the nar-
row beach got crowded and people moved out to find their own
space. Inevitably, some of them started rounding the bend and
approached the Spanish Banks beach, "shocking the general public." In 1983 police arrested eight people for nudity on the
Foreshore area of the beach, but the Crown dropped the charges.
Attorney General Garde Gardom declared that "skinny dipping in
a moderate sense is something that has been a bit of a way of life
in Canada." In a two-and-a-half-hour meeting between the
Director of Policy and Legal Services and the Wreck Beach
Preservation Society on 19 July 1984, the Attorney General's office
made clear that they "were not inclined to consent to prosecutions
for nudity on Wreck Beach."[11]

There is more than nudity to Wreck Beach; there is also a
unique ambience that attracts people from near and far. They sun,
they swim, read, play frisbee or volleyball, enjoy the live entertainment offered by wandering musicians and jugglers, and take
in the rich human kaleidoscope that passes along the beach.[12]

There are serpents in this Garden of Eden, however. On a public beach where nudity is optional rather than obligatory there are
always gawkers—the "perverts sitting in the bushes"—who ironically were first attracted to Wreck Beach by the 1970 Nude-In.
They have been joined by more brazen "peekers" who walk the
beach with cameras at the ready. The heavily wooded cliffs and
isolated breakwaters offer seclusion for "couples engaging in sex-

ual activities." And the "gay section" along the Fraser River has been the site of "strange sexual doings."[13]

Another nuisance to beachgoers are the myriad vendors pushing materialism at people who come to Wreck Beach to escape it. The downside of this free enterprise response to market demand is that the beach is strewn with bottles, cans, wrappers, plastic and styrofoam containers, cigarette butts, and the occasional "hot pink condom." Alcohol and drugs are another problem for beach-goers and police. And until the GVRD Parks Board took over there were no washroom facilities for people or pets. All these things detract from the original natural appeal of the beach, and drive some people away.[14]

In December 1988 Premier Bill Vander Zalm announced the formation of Pacific Spirit Regional Park, a huge new urban park that would encompass all of Wreck Beach. In April 1989 the Greater Vancouver Regional District (GVRD) took over control of Wreck Beach and the University Endowment Lands. This offered beachgoers the promise of basic park facilities—drinking fountains, washrooms, waste containers—for the first time. One year later, on 16 May 1990, the GVRD Park Committee accepted a staff report which recommended official "clothing optional" status for Wreck Beach based on "historic use," the isolated location of the beach, and the Attorney General's policy regarding public nudity. The full Park Committee "established the first official clothing optional beach in a Canadian regional park" on 16 October 1991. On 30 October, the GVRD Board of Directors ratified the Park Committee's action. Canada had its first legal nude beach.[15]

At first glance the Prairies might seem unpromising territory for nude beaches, but Alberta was home to a legally tolerated free beach in the 1970s and Saskatchewan is the site of a significant court ruling on skinny-dipping, while Manitoba's many lakes and fine sandy beaches provide innumerable isolated locations for individual and group sunbathing.

Canyon Valley Park (CVP) was the brainchild of two Alberta

members of the Western Canadian Sunbathing Association (WCSA) who found they shared a common perspective on nudism and on the need for a greater range of nudist options than just the traditional clubs. A park open to the general public seemed to be an appropriate alternative. The Canyon Valley partners contacted various government agencies, including the solicitor general, the minister of tourism, and the minister of culture, sport, and recreation. They all proved willing to work with Canyon Valley Facilities and regarded the park as a test case to determine the demand for, and attitudes towards, nude recreation in Alberta.[16]

In 1972 CVF obtained a mile-long stretch of land on the south shore of Wizard Lake in central Alberta, about 40 miles southwest of Edmonton. Canyon Valley operated as a privately owned nudist park. Unlike WCSA clubs, Canyon Valley did not require its patrons to belong to CVF, the WCSA, or to any other organization, but simply recorded license plate numbers, charged a gate fee for admission, and required that children be accompanied by parents. The solicitor general instructed the RCMP to tolerate nude swimming, canoeing, and sailing at Canyon Valley and to ignore unwarranted complaints. The curious snuck up through the woods or paid admission, even though they were "just coming to look," but these were minor distractions. In the words of the CVF Public Relations Officer, "we are a local curiosity but we have very good local public relations."[17]

In 1972 more than 600 people visited Canyon Valley's 160 acres to swim, canoe, sail, fish, sunbathe, camp—and hike (the beach was down a 200-foot cliff). Some people looking for the Wizard Lake Waterski Club wound up at Canyon Valley by mistake, but later on skiers ran down the lake to visit—as many as 700 on one memorable day—and several eventually joined landed clubs in Edmonton and Calgary.[18]

Despite the relative success of Canyon Valley, both partners felt compelled to end the operation after two more seasons because of the practical difficulties of running the park from separate offices in Edmonton and Calgary. In 1974 a Helios couple took over the site, built a new access road, and renamed it Conjuring Park. The western portion of the land was sold to an Edmonton couple, not involved with Helios or Conjuring Park, who reserved it for a small circle of friends who remained "somewhat independent of strict ASA guidelines." Conjuring Park continued to operate for several more years, though with diminishing attendance, as visitors grew discouraged with a nude beach that was sheltered from the sun all day. When Helios found its own camp closer to Edmonton, Conjuring Park closed.[19]

Around the time that Conjuring Park disappeared, Karl Wilde opened Alberta's second free beach resort on a pond called Falken Lake. Wilde, a native of Germany who had worked in Ontario for several years before moving to Alberta, bought the 150-acre site in 1980 and opened the Golden Acres Nudist Camp the next year. But the camp quickly collapsed when prairie men overreacted to the naked women. Wilde reorganized his operation and reopened it in 1983 as Wildesheim Resort, although his advance publicity aroused the ire of Bible-belt farmers.[20]

Seven hundred people visited Wildesheim in 1983, at $30 per couple, and Wilde devised ambitious plans for a multi-million-dollar complex on the "European resort model." For 1984 he planned to lease plots for $2,500 and charge user fees of $350. But the plans remained pipedreams. The second season was less successful than the first, with only a few dozen visitors per weekend willing to drive to Red Deer to spend the day sitting around a "dredged slough." Although an emergency appeal to nudist clubs in Edmonton and Calgary brought 130 sunbathers in late July, 1984 proved to be the last season and Wilde lost the camp to foreclosure.[21]

The lakes and rivers of Saskatchewan also attract nudists—so much so that Bare Ass Beach in Saskatoon became the occasion for a definitive ruling on the legality of skinnydipping in Canada. When three young men were arrested for nude swimming in the South Saskatchewan River in 1975, Mr. Justice MacPherson ruled in their favor.

It cannot be an offense to swim in the nude at a lonely place in Canada in summer. That is part of the pleasure of summer in Canada, particularly to young males. If somebody comes along unexpectedly or if the swimmer misjudged the loneliness of the place the act cannot suddenly become criminal. . . .

The present accused were not disorderly. There was no indecency or immorality. That was their lawful excuse.[22]

In Manitoba two large and relatively isolated lakes, along with numerous smaller lakes and rivers, have all beckoned naturists to improvise their own free beaches. The Manitoba Outdoor Club did nothing but visit secluded lakeshore and riverine beaches during its first decade, and even with Winnipeg's growth there remain many uninhabited areas nearby for sunning and swimming. Some of these sites, such as Patricia Beach, have acquired a local reputation and attract a regular group of visitors, with public and media tolerance, as reflected by "Miss Lonelyhearts" in the *Winnipeg Sun*.[23]

In 1998 some complaints arose over another beach at Beaconia. That summer several nearby residents wandered onto the traditionally nude section of the beach and claimed to be offended by "indecent exposure" and "public gay sex." A public battle erupted in town council meetings between naturists and environmentalists who wanted to enjoy the beach naturally, on the one hand, and locals who wanted to tear up the beach with ATVs, on the other hand. The council—presumably after being advised on the limits of local jurisdiction over crown land—decided not to prosecute. The beach itself is sufficiently remote from "family" areas that no one (at least no one on foot) need be offended by nudity.[24]

Ontario possesses hundreds of thousands of inland lakes, hundreds of miles of Great Lakes shoreline, and countless rivers which invite swimming, sunning, canoeing, and sailing *au naturel*. Despite its relatively large population and high urban density, most of these areas remain open to naturist activity—but with discretion, for unlike virtually every other province, Ontario did not grant official tolerance to nude beaches until the end of the century, although Leo Bernier, Tory Minister for Natural Resources, came surprisingly close in 1972 when he commented that "although I must admit that nudism in our parks is one of the more novel uses of the system, I can foresee a vast number of diversified uses of outdoor recreation land in the future."[25]

In Toronto, a large metropolitan area "blessed with some very lovely river valleys," the Don and the Humber were major venues for skinny-dipping from the 1890s to the early 1950s.

> It is a beautiful sight on a sunny afternoon to stand on the edge of the hill, high above the river, and see the nude bodies of many carefree youths, splashing in the water, or lying on the banks, soaking in the sunshine.[26]

When Hurricane Hazel ruined "the best spots in the Don Valley" in 1954, bathers moved to the Lake Ontario shoreline at Cherry Beach, Sunnyside Beach, and Hanlan's Point—"the most popular public nudist beach in the Toronto area," albeit heavily policed. In later years the Scarborough Bluffs, with their difficult cliffside access, provided sunbathing that is relatively secluded.[27]

In 1997 TNT!MEN, a Toronto gay nudist club, collected signatures on a petition to set up a nude beach at Hanlan's Point. When it submitted a brief to Toronto City Council in April 1999 their lawyer noted the popularity of nude beaches around the world, particularly the Canadian precedents at Wreck Beach and Meech Lake. He also recounted the history of legalized nudity at Hanlan's Point from 1894 until 1930, noted the chronic underuse of an attractive and convenient beach, and argued that legalization would be good for Toronto's "world class" self-image and would quickly pay for itself ($5,000 in start-up costs and $400,000 in additional ferry revenues). On 12 May City Council accepted the proposal on the recommendation of the Economic Development Committee, in time for TNT!MEN to host a celebration on the beach over Victoria Day weekend, featuring a club member appropriately attired as Queen Victoria and looking quite amused. Two years later city council voted to extend the life and the dimensions of the free beach area, given its proven success.[28]

Along the Great Lakes there are free beach areas at Sandbanks Provincial Park in Prince Edward County, at Sherkston Cliffs near Port Colborne on the Niagara Peninsula, and at Pinery Park on Lake Huron that have been used by naturists for decades.[29]

In southwest Ontario nudism almost achieved the legal tolerance called for by Mr Bernier. At a spring meeting of the Kent County Tourist Association in 1976 Pearl Wortner, co-owner of the Sunny Glades club in Bothwell, asked her fellow board members to "consider nude bathing on a specified public beach within the county" because "a 'bathing suit optional' beach in Kent County would bring tourists and the tourist dollar." Other board members asked her to present a formal proposal at the next meeting. Wortner settled on Rondeau Park as the most appropriate location—possibly because of the long tradition of skinnydipping at Rondeau, Erieau, and Sleepy Hollow—with the beach to be managed by the Thames Valley Conservation Authority.[30] But she had not reckoned with the good folks of Kent County, who complained that "the new generation wears few enough clothes—patches, holes, ragged, faded and bare navels" and who noted that "even in the garden of Eden they at least tried to cover themselves with a fig leaf." The whole episode was summed up by the *Sarnia Observer* in an editorial: "Kent County is not particularly in the vanguard of open-mindedness on the practice of nudism."[31]

Neighboring Essex County is home to one of the most popular nude beaches in Ontario at Point Pelee. The beach on the east side of the Point has been used for nude sunbathing for half a century. But in the 1970s, when members of Sunny Glades approached the park superintendent about sunbathing, he informed them that "Point Pelee National Park, as its name implies, is a National Park set aside for use by all people of Canada for their benefit, education and enjoyment"—as long as they aren't sunbathing: "this would probably result in charges being laid against the offending person or persons."[32]

In the mid-1980s park officials decided to crack down on nude sunbathing after receiving an alarming "two to three complaints" during the year. They posted a sign notifying bathers of park regulations regarding appropriate formal attire. Despite the isolated location of the beach officials levied fines, evicted some offenders, and arrested others. Eventually, the typically bureaucratic policy of out-of-sight, out-of-mind prevailed, and nudists simply moved down the road to other conservation areas.[33]

Inland lakes throughout Ontario are popular for nude sailing and nude canoeing. Although not all canoeists are nudists, most enjoy nature and tolerate others who enjoy nature, making for "a greater freedom to practice the nude lifestyle in the wilderness than one might suppose." Virtually all of Ontario off the beaten path is safe for discreet camping, hiking, and canuding. Among the areas favored for nude canoeing are Algonquin Park, Quetico Park, the Rideau Lakes, Temagami, and scattered lakes throughout the province, including McCrae Lake north of Toronto, where naturists can enjoy "lots of bays and rocky points to camp on. Some of the campsites even have sandy beaches."[34]

Boaters also are "taking off everything to gain this feeling of freedom." Lake Simcoe accommodates scores of nude sailors, although naturists tend to congregate off the south and east shores of Georgina Island and around Thorah Island, where nudity is tolerated by boaters and by police.[35]

Georgian Bay has been used for nude sailing since the 1940s. On the west side of the Bay, White Cloud Island off the Bruce Peninsula has a long tradition of nude sailing, swimming, and sunning. In the 1950s the CSA group leader from Owen Sound offered a "nudist cruise through the beautiful 30,000 islands"— before moving to Florida. Today "many more boaters enjoy nude freedom" in the same area.[36]

In the national capital, competing with the better-known and more popular Meech Lake across the river in Quebec, several secluded spots along the Ottawa and Rideau rivers have been used for nude sunbathing, including Hogs Back Falls at Carleton University. For that matter, the entire Rideau Canal system is open to nude boating and sailing, provided the nudity is not blatantly visible to landlubbers (or to sunfish).[37]

Meech Lake is probably the most celebrated beach in eastern Canada. The Gatineau Park area in Quebec has attracted nude sunbathers for decades. They gather at the Carbide Willson Mill, in an isolated corner of Meech Lake. Periodically, authorities attempted to discourage practitioners by hauling them away to be fingerprinted and warned, but they kept coming back—so much so that in 1984 the National Capital Commission (NCC), which has jurisdiction over federal parks in the Ottawa-Hull area, decided that regulation was the better part of valor. In June the NCC announced that it would tolerate nude sunbathing in one section of Gatineau Park: the Carbide Willson Mill on Meech Lake. Though not a pleasant environment—"the dirtiest, ugliest place they could find"—it was better than nothing. "For many Ottawa residents, it provides an ideal escape back to normalcy, away from the nonsense and lunacy that permeates the nation's capital these days."[38]

At the very moment that the NCC grudgingly set aside one small area for nudists it cracked down on nudism elsewhere in the park. On Sunday, 17 June, Kevin Hogan went out to the park and spread his towel on a part of the beach just outside the designated area. A patrol boat happened by, and a park officer warned people to dress. Hogan refused because he had not seen any of the new signs. Arguing that invisibility of the law was no excuse, the rangers arrested Hogan for violating article 18 of the NCC regulations, which states that "no one may utter blasphemous or indecent words nor conduct himself in an offensive manner on the grounds of the Commission."[39]

On 9 January 1985, provincial court judge Jules Barrière of the district of Hull acquitted Hogan. In an eleven-page statement the judge declared that nudity is a matter of criminal law and cannot be governed by NCC regulations. Moreover, he even criticized the NCC for setting aside one area for sunbathing. "It seems that the Commission has even taken upon itself the right to permit the committing of a criminal offense by announcing that it would tolerate nudity on a certain part of its territory." Although Hogan was acquitted, it was not so much a victory for nudism as a ruling against one tactic used by the NCC. Other tactics remained.[40]

In spring of 1986 the NCC announced that for the coming summer season it would invoke the Criminal Code and attempt to prosecute all nude sunbathers anywhere in the park. But the Quebec Provincial Police repeated its position that it would lay charges only if citizens complained in writing and agreed to testify in court; they would not respond to anonymous complaints. In order to persuade citizens to do their duty the NCC prepared a pamphlet for park visitors on how to arrest a nudist. The *Ottawa Citizen* commiserated with the beleaguered commission: "if only the NCC could find a little old lady willing to patrol the Gatineau and lodge complaints whenever she found too much skin."[41]

Needless to say, the little old ladies did not choose to clamber over the rocks and through the woods to search for naked people, and the NCC and the nudists remained at odds over the propriety of nude sunbathing in the secluded Carbide Willson Mill area. In 1997 and 1998 the nudists started posting their own signs to advise passers-by that "you may encounter nude sunbathers." While reluctant to sanction a designated clothing-optional area, an NCC spokesperson admitted in 1999 that "we don't have the authority to permit or prohibit or enforce activities under the criminal code." Today the Carbide Willson Mill area continues to be "frequented by up to a hundred naturists on a typical warm summer weekend."[42]

Quebec's decades-old skinnydipping tradition, combined with the increasingly freer social atmosphere after 1960, encouraged more and more people to practice "wild nudism." As they did so, a number of locations along rivers and lakes acquired local reputations for nude bathing. In Quebec, as in Ontario, naturism is compatible with canoe-camping. One naturist who joined a weekend trip reported that canoeists were quite sympathetic to naturism and often swam nude at rest stops.[43]

By the late 1970s the FQN counted nearly forty sites in Quebec and Vermont that were used by naturists. Few of these locations were officially tolerated, and this created the ever-present risk of prosecution. Over the years, some of these beach areas were raided, and charges were laid after complaints about nudity. In 1980 the QPP raided Cap Rouge on the St. Lawrence near Quebec City and arrested twenty-nine men in an incident which became a *cause célèbre*, at least on the pages of the *Journal de Québec*, which reported it under the headline, "Sex orgy or sunbath?" In July 1986 the QPP, acting on local complaints, arrested thirteen people at St. Jean de Matha, and in August police in Montreal arrested fourteen people on the Ile des Soeurs in the St. Lawrence.[44]

The first legally recognized nude beach in Quebec was at Pointe Taillon on the north shore of Lake St. Jean. Its reputation grew over the years, so that by 1980 average weekend attendance topped three hundred people of all ages. But when the corporate owner of the land, Alcan, decided to turn it over for development as a provincial park, the Ministry of Recreation announced that nude sunbathing would no longer be permitted. Local nudists immediately organized and contacted the FQN, which submitted a brief to the ministry requesting continued tolerance for the tradition of nudity and suggesting the demarcation of a designated clothing optional zone marked by signs. In December 1981, the local office of the ministry responded by stating that a government facility could not favor one segment of the public over another but that, after obtaining legal advice, it had decided to "tolerate the presence of naturists on the beach at Pointe Taillon."[45]

The FQN celebrated its victory: "for the first time in Canada you are officially welcome as nudists on a public beach." For the most part, nudists appreciated and enjoyed the beach at Taillon.

> It was the nicest free beach I've ever visited, with a greater number of users than any other except Vancouver's Wreck Beach. There was a better balance of the sexes and a good family ambience.[46]

After two enjoyable summers with thousands of visitors to the beach, the ministry had a change of heart and informed the FQN that it would not renew the arrangement. Albert Courville, regional director of the FQN, hastily arranged a meeting with officials in May 1984, and they agreed to permit the 100 meter beach to continue for that season. The ministry also invited the Federation to participate in public hearings the following year regarding the final transformation of Pointe Taillon into a provincial park.[47]

Several organizations supported the FQN at the hearings, including the CEGEP at St Felicien, the Regional Recreation Council, the Regional Tourist Association, and the Regroupement Loisirs Québec. Two geographers from the University of Quebec at Chicoutimi also supported the nude beach on the basis that nudity was an established tradition at the beach, that nudists came from all over the province, that nudists are taxpayers and have the right to expect use of some public facilities, that nudism is an increasingly popular pastime, and that naturism is supportive of the natural beach at Taillon.[48]

The ministry chose to accept the opposing representations from the local citizens and to discontinue its toleration of the nude beach. But the FQN did not give up, and in 1987 it was able to negotiate another temporary arrangement with the ministry to allow sunbathing in exchange for increased supervision of the beach by the FQN, a pledge that the naturists would dress if other groups approached their beach, and a promise to maintain a low profile. This policy expired with the transfer of the local official to the boonies, but nude bathing remains popular at Pointe Taillon, though on a reduced scale from the 1980s.[49]

One of the most popular and accessible free beaches near Montreal was Oka Beach in Paul Sauvé Park. In the early 1980s

nudists found toleration from local officials, who directed newcomers to the nude area of the beach. In 1982 the FQN presented
a brief to the minister of recreation at public hearings on the future
of Oka Beach. The FQN argued for the health benefits of naturism,
particularly on beaches where the sun, air, and water combined
with the "calming effect" of social nudity to provide "physical and
mental equilibrium." The ministry was not convinced, and argued
that legal recognition would be premature because public opinion
was not prepared to accept such action.[50]

During the following years nudists continued to frequent Oka
Beach and reported *de facto* tolerance at the park. In 1984
Montreal papers commented on the nude beach and on the
acceptance of nudists by non-nudists, who "chose the spot
because the main beach area is too crowded, too noisy, and lit-
tered with garbage." In 1985 the FQN promoted World Nudism
Day at Oka. In recent years park officials have made a more concerted effort to advise visitors of the law, and have made some
arrests. But this approach backfired; "the more signs, the more
nudists." Oka continues to attract hundreds of nudists on weekends. The chief factor limiting its popularity now is pollution,
along with "exhibitionists and voyeurs." Recently the FQN
staged a clean-up day at Oka on World Naturism Day, earning the
appreciation of the minister of the environment. The police, too,
are more sympathetic, pledging to arrest only persons engaging in
indecent behavior, not sunbathing naturists. "The majority of the
textiles tolerate and even enjoy the sight of nude freedom, but
some of them continue to hassle us verbally and always try to
chase us away."[51]

A unique experiment in operating a commercial free beach on
the Alberta pattern occurred in the Eastern Townships during the
mid-1980s. In 1985 Marc Fournier formed the Plein Soleil Estrie
(PSE) company to operate nude beaches in the region. The first
location was Key Brook, near Sherbrooke. It was a propitious
choice since the area had a naturist tradition dating back fifty
years. But the following year, when PSE leased Coconut Beach on
Lake Massawippi (which also had a tradition of skinny dipping),

the reaction was different. Local townspeople compiled a petition against the beach, signed by 440 people.[52]

What made this nude beach controversial was the fact that the ultimate landlord of the property was Canadian Pacific Railway, and CPR opposed Plein Soleil. In July CPR police raided the beach, demanded identification from everyone present, and took photographs. CPR announced that it would seek an injunction against PSE in order to "restore to the residents of West Hatley free access to their beach." CPR spokesman Ralph Wilson claimed that the company had no opposition to nudism but simply wanted to be a good neighbor. On 15 July 1986, the St François District Court granted the injunction. Although the ruling affected only one of Plein Soleil's operations, the time and money involved in this legal battle discouraged Fournier and his members, and PSE drifted apart. Only Key Brook remained open, under new management.[53]

On the east coast the Atlantic provinces are surrounded by relatively warm ocean water and wrapped by fine sandy beaches, all making naturism an attractive prospect for this thinly populated region, while in New Brunswick and Nova Scotia rivers and lakes offer secluded venues for swimming and sunning. Newfoundland even offers the opportunity to "sit on the hill, au naturel, and admire the icebergs and the clean air. It is wonderful." At Kelly's Beach in Kouchibouguac Park in New Brunswick and at Blooming Point Beach on Prince Edward Island there are "families with children, couples, singles, those young and old, all enjoying the ambience the concept of naturism embraces."[54]

The most famous of the free beaches in Atlantic Canada is Crystal Crescent Beach, near Halifax. For years Haligonians gathered at the third cove on Crystal Crescent, and the local tourist office provided maps and directions for newcomers. But in August 1990 the RCMP patrolled the beach for the first time after receiving complaints about "perverts," and claimed that "we got an eyeful." The hundred or more sunbathers blamed the action on the fact that land adjoining the beach was up for sale. Media coverage was sympathetic; one reporter even joined the nudists.

Although the matter was referred to the attorney general, beach-goers organized themselves as the Bluenose Naturist Club and stood off the threat to their beach, with support from the Federation of Canadian Naturists and from the International Naturist Federation. They now meet year-round, using rented indoor pools in winter and conducting regular beach sweeps in summer like their more famous counterparts on Wreck Beach.[55]

CHAPTER TEN

A House Divided

The history of the Canadian Sunbathing Association is the history of the rise and fall of Ray Connett in the minds and hearts of Canadian nudists. In May 1946 Connett contacted the American Sunbathing Association to resume his writing for *Sunshine & Health* and to announce plans to organize Vancouver-area nudists. Then in July Connett suggested "something much more important"—the formation of a Canadian Sunbathing Association. Throughout 1947 Connett and a handful of others prepared for the big day. There were anxious moments over the question of incorporation—was it necessary? federally or provincially?—which they settled by shelving the matter until the association grew large enough to warrant incorporation (and the $300 fee required). But at long last Connett could write, "the time has come!"[1]

On Saturday and Sunday, 18-19 October 1947, two score enthusiasts, escaping a threatened transit strike but not a drenching dose of "Vancouver sunshine," met in the Arcadian Hall in Vancouver to establish an organization "to foster and promote the practice of social nudism." On the agenda were the name and constitution of the organization, election of officers, membership and dues, and the relationship between the national organization and local clubs.[2]

When the group assembled, Ray Connett called for the election of a convention chairman. This responsibility fell to Roy McKague, former leader of the Sun Air Freedom Lovers and now a member of the Van Tans. Then Don, a lifelong nudist from British Columbia's Galiano Island, introduced a motion "to inaugurate a Canadian Sunbathing Association." Ray Connett had prepared a draft constitution for discussion based on the models of

the ASA and the Central Sunbathing Association, a regional affiliate of the ASA. In this way the three-member committee—Don,
Hazel McKague, and Roy Ramey—were able to present a finished
draft the next day, allowing for an evening dance hosted by the
Van Tans.[3]

The CSA was set up as a national organization composed of
individual and group members of adult age (21). Dues were set to
favor club members, but all CSA members were to receive *Sunny
Trails* magazine—the "official organ of the CSA," which would publish official news as well as proposals to be discussed at the annual
conventions. The national executive board consisted of a president,
a secretary, and a treasurer (all elected annually), and four directors
or members at large elected for two-year terms, two each year. The
intention was that two would be from the west and two from the
east, since at the time there were only two established clubs in
Canada. A regional convention in one part of the country would
precede the national convention in the other part. The executive
board would act to implement decisions made at the conventions,
which would combine votes on proposals published in *Sunny Trails*,
although constitutional amendments required a two-thirds majority
of votes at the conventions. All in all it was "a dream . . . come true,"
one that "marked a real beginning for nudism in Canada."[4]

Once the CSA was formed in 1947 Connett pushed publicity
for all he could by constantly keeping nudism before the public in
a straightforward but never straightlaced manner. Connett and
the CSA were responsible for sympathetic articles over the years in
such national publications as *Macleans*, *Time*, and *Liberty*. In later
years radio and TV were utilized as well. This "carefully cultivated publicity" made nudism and the CSA accepted and respected
by local officials, the police, the media, and public opinion.[5]

Another successful publicity effort was the CSA booth at the
Pacific National Exhibition for several years during the mid-1950s.
This was largely the brainchild of Rex Craig, publicity director for
the CSA in 1955. The booth itself was decorated in the green and
gold colors of the CSA and featured a large back panel containing

club pictures and press clippings. "We almost had to shoo the nudists out of the booth to make room for non-nudist visitors." Volunteers handed out thousands of pamphlets and brochures to people "who might never see a nudist magazine." At least one visitor was impressed enough to write to *Sunbathing for Health* later: "I first became interested in your organization when I picked up some folders at the PNE in 1954."[6]

The CSA was less successful in its attempt to screen the first modern nudist film, *Garden of Eden*. In 1954 Walter Bibo and Excelsior Pictures produced a movie at the Lake Como Club near Tampa, Florida, which depicted some non-nudists who accidentally wind up in a nudist club. Their initial moralistic reaction to nudity turns to approval when they see how friendly, innocent, and natural the nudists are.[7]

The *American Sunbather* magazine predicted that *Garden of Eden* "will make nudist history and history in the cinema world." Actually, it made more history in the world of film censorship, since state censor boards throughout the United States tried to ban the film. All attempts were defeated, but often only after lengthy court battles. In Canada, however, authorities were more successful in banning the film because their jurisdiction was less subject to public scrutiny and legal appeal. (The 1933 film *Elysia* was still banned in Canada in the 1950s.)[8]

Trouble started when Bibo shipped a promotional photo album to the CSA and it was held up by "the severe censorship of the postal authorities in eastern Canada." The film itself was delayed by the Ontario film censor, "who is afraid to give the picture the green light" unless Bibo or the CSA could provide authoritative testimonials on the merits of the film from irreproachable public figures. Connett, out in Vancouver, tried to persuade Bibo and the would-be Canadian distributor, Cardinal Films, to submit the film to the B.C. censor board first because it had assured Connett that "viewing audiences in the west are much more tolerant and stable." But Cardinal Films preferred to target Ontario because of the larger market, and lost out in both markets. When the movie played in Buffalo, Ontario nudists organized cross-border freedom excursions to see it, and Sun Valley Gardens distributed its club brochure in the souvenir program. But *Garden of Eden* remained banned in Canada for years afterwards.[9]

The most practical work which the CSA carried out was its mandate "to encourage the formation of new clubs." Ray Connett published articles every month in *Sunbathing for Health* and *Sunshine & Health* to reach the general public. People who became interested wrote in to Connett, who reprinted their letters on his "Reader's Page," or they wrote to a specific club or group and Connett forwarded the letters after sending out an array of pro-motional material for the CSA, *Sunny Trails*, and the magazine subscription service operated by Mildred Connett. This routine helped promote the growth of virtually every nudist club in Canada, but once a "group" became a "club" with land and a solid membership base it started to resent outside interference from Connett and the CSA. The clubs criticized the procedure whereby an applicant living near a club had to write to that club by way of a magazine published in Toronto which forwarded the letter to the CSA in Vancouver which eventually passed it on to the club.[10]

A second issue that got the clubs "fed up with the CSA" was the publication of club news in *Sunny Trails* magazine. Connett adopted the practice of extracting juicy tidbits from all letters sent to him for any reason and publishing them in his magazine or in one of his columns in *Sunbathing for Health*. Club owners and prospective members objected to having their dirty laundry aired in public, particularly given the low caliber of many of the readers of both magazines.[11]

Another perennial sore point between the CSA and the clubs was the association's openness to single applicants, with "no strict weeding out." Anyone who paid dues got accepted, and then the CSA insisted, as it did at the 1948 convention, that clubs should accept its members without the customary interviews and screen-ing, even though Connett agreed that "most of the CSA members are 'odds and sods' who cannot get into a club or haven't bothered to join one." And Connett also acknowledged that the CSA's "mysterious screening process" was "practically non-existent," but he justified this sham by his belief "that 99 out of every 100 people can become good nudists." The only exceptions that he recognized were social misfits and the "sexually aberrant." Unfortunately, not only applicants but even some CSA district organizers were "sexually aberrant," such as one Ontario representative who was blacklisted in 1952 when the CSA received a letter that he wrote to an applicant—"My darling Jimmy"—which contained irrefutable proof of his proclivities.[12]

The heart of the problem was that the CSA, as a "2-bit paper organization" in Vancouver, simply lacked the resources to monitor its own officials, let alone the rank and file. Connett accepted sight unseen anyone "who writes a nice letter," and this procedure occasionally backfired, particularly in relations with eastern clubs. When the CSA representative was a member of another local—and therefore rival—club, the potential for acrimony was high. When that representative found himself at odds in his own club as well as with other clubs, an explosion was inevitable.[13]

The most dramatic case in point involved Bob Babcock from Norhaven and the Sunglades Club in Toronto. Sunglades had a longstanding quarrel with Bob ever since the club formed against his advice: "our province . . . can hardly do justice to the one club it already has, so what hope can a new one have?" Over the years Bob continued to rile Sunglades by questioning its elitist admission policies. He asked Sunglades to send him all the applications that it did not accept so that he could contact them on behalf of his club. Ironically, by the time Sunglades forwarded the letters to him Bob was no longer club secretary and was about to resign as CSA eastern director. It was particularly his status as director that upset Sunglades, because they thought him unfit for the position. In addition, several Sunglades members had personal quarrels with Bob during visits to Norhaven. One, Cedric, tried to arrange for a private access road and cottage site on Otter Lake, for which Bob had him expelled from the club.[14]

In the spring of 1952 Bob mailed a negative that he had received from a friend in the United States to a photographer friend in Toronto who belonged to both clubs, and who in turn showed it to the Sunglades club photographer, who gave it to the club president, Ken, who found it "INDECENT BEYOND DESCRIPTION." In his capacity as CSA eastern secretary Ken wrote on CSA letterhead (the CSA always claimed he wrote on club stationery) to Vancouver, calling for "drastic action" in view of Bob's "keen interest in this type of 'art'." He then left for a six-week tour of England, and the new Sunglades president, Dennis, refused to forward the negative to Vancouver. Without evidence the CSA could do nothing.[15]

Then Sunglades received another package from North Bay containing several pictures (prints rather than negatives) and a typed letter signed "Bob." This time Bob vehemently denied any involvement. It is true that this package was sent to the club's general address, whereas Bob had sent the first set directly to the couple. Since it came so soon after the first incident, Bob suspected a "frame-up" or worse: "who ever is responsible not only wanted me out of Norhaven but also wanted me scared out of the whole movement." It was clear that this second package arrived at a time when both clubs were still upset about the first incident, so anyone aware of that crisis knew that "the time was right for his dirty work."[16]

Dennis suggested an alternative scenario. He argued that, since the first incident had split Sunglades apart and had led to Ken's resignation, and since there was a rival club forming in Toronto, John, the organizer of the Roving Suntans, was responsible. Later that year Dennis reported that John had described the pictures to a new Sunglades applicant, and since only a few people had seen the photos after they arrived, this could mean only that John had seen it before it was sent, and had therefore sent it himself in an effort to break Sunglades rather than Norhaven.[17]

But there were problems with this interpretation, too. John had first contacted the CSA in July, a month *after* the second package arrived in Toronto. Moreover, he didn't seem to be the type to mastermind a plot to destroy two well-established clubs and take over Ontario. "This man has very little notion of what is involved in his rather optimistic plan for a club without perhaps having the personality, nor character to see the thing through properly. . . . He might be a reasonably good member, but not likely to prove a good leader."[18]

There was another possibility: a new club, opening in Hamilton, that posed a more serious threat to Sunglades. Jack, a former CSA group leader in Saskatoon, moved to Hamilton and took charge of the group there. He moved quickly and forcefully to set up an active club, bought 28 acres of land, gathered ten couples, and watched as Sunglades lost its land west of Toronto in the spring. The Hamilton Sunbathing Club graciously invited the homeless Sunglades members to use their camp, and to attend their "official opening" on 3 August 1952.[19]

Jack also happened to be president of the Ontario chapter of the Society of Natural Living, "a notorious picture trading outfit." The CSA had already had a run-in with Jack when he asked to buy "photos of camp activity," offered to develop pictures for CSA members, and sought to advertise for the Canadian Society of Natural Living in *Sunny Trails*. All these requests were refused. By spring 1952 his reputation was such that the CSA enlisted Bob at Norhaven—who had his own connections with picture traders—to investigate Jack and his club. In January 1953 the CSA board reviewed the evidence and concluded that it "places him unquestionably as a pornographic picture trader of the worst type and suggests that his own moral and intra-group conduct is highly questionable." Since Jack made repeated attempts to lure Sungladers to his club, and since the Society of Natural Living included Toronto members who had been rejected by Sunglades, it is entirely possible that he or someone connected with him was responsible for the second picture incident. In any case, there were no further incidents between Norhaven and Sunglades after the CSA dropped both Jack in Hamilton and John in Toronto.[20]

By the end of 1952 the CSA executive in Vancouver was fed up with the complaints and problems of easterners, and decided to call their bluff. In a "swan song" in January 1953 Ray informed prominent eastern leaders about western opinion regarding the future of the CSA.

> Reg [Nicholls] hits close to home when he asks if Western CSA officials are sick of hearing Eastern troubles and scandals and back-biting, so that they neglect to answer letters. Western CSA officials are sick, period. Bewildered. This particular Western CSA official is so sick of the series of nauseating bilge that has come out of the East that he wonders whether it has all been worthwhile.[21]

Connett was indeed burned out by 1953. Writing three columns per month in *Sunbathing for Health* and all of *Sunny Trails*, in addition to occasional columns for *Sunshine & Health*, on top of serving as secretary and work supervisor at the Van Tan Club and later at the Sunny Trails Club, while also organizing the CSA and serving as its perennial secretary, not to mention holding down a full-time job at the post office and moving from one home to another in postwar Vancouver while trying to keep up the semblance of family life: this all brought him too close to the breaking point. Not surprisingly, he sometimes snapped at clubs, leaders, and officials, and they snapped back. It was bad enough when he quarrelled with west-coast nudists, most of whom he knew and saw regularly. But when he dealt with easterners sight unseen it was easy for both sides to fly off the handle. The Quetans crisis simply added salt to the wounds. Connett and the entire "Connett-controlled CSA" (Couture's term) wanted out, and they proposed to hand the whole show over to the east in 1953.[22]

Everything was ready for the passing of the torch, but the east blew its big chance by scheduling the national convention during peak forest fire season, and rangers forced a last-minute cancellation. The West had already voted in August to affiliate with the ASA and to elect easterners to national office. When the eastern convention was cancelled, a mail ballot was conducted on both proposals. After several nominees declined to stand, Albert

"Thornton" of Norhaven and Albert "Taylor" of Sunglades became national president and secretary, respectively. Two other easterners became regional secretaries: Mel in Ontario and Marcus Meed in the Maritimes. The national treasurer (Audrey) and publicity director (Ray) were westerners. Ray also served as western regional secretary. Affiliation with the ASA was approved overwhelmingly.[23]

The question of affiliation with the ASA hovered over the CSA even before it was a gleam in the founding father's eye. When Connett first proposed a Canadian organization to ASA officials he assured them that this Canadian association "would of course be affiliated with you and subsidiary to the ASA." In response, the ASA promised that "with your publicity, educational, and organizational program we should be glad to cooperate 100%." But on the question of affiliation—"an excellent suggestion, to be sure"—they offered only to consider the proposal. In September the Executive Director of the ASA, Ilsley "Uncle Danny" Boone, an ordained minister and self-promoter in the Elmer Gantry style, flew to Vancouver to meet with Connett and the Van Tans, who were debating club affiliation with the ASA. While Boone earnestly pitched affiliation to the club, he advised against it for the future Canadian association.

> No, he said, the Canadian nudist movement must stand firmly on its own two feet or it will never stand at all. No, uncle Danny stressed that we could look to the ASA for every cooperation as brothers, or much as Canada itself looks to the U.S.A., but never as a subsidiary to it.[24]

Unfortunately for Uncle Danny, not everyone in America felt the same way as his "starry eyed" disciple in Vancouver. In 1951 rebels opposed to Boone's one-man rule ousted his hand-picked board and voted in their own candidates. Boone contested this action, and the Supreme Court of New Jersey placed the ASA in receivership until a new convention in 1952 drafted a more democratic constitution. This document of course precluded Boone's personal control, and he left to form a rival organization, the National Nudist Council.[25]

The new ASA wasted no time in asking the CSA to reconsider affiliation. Norval Packwood, the ASA executive director who succeeded Uncle Danny, argued that "it is becoming more and more apparent that the interlocking of activities between the Canadian and American Sunbathing organizations is fast reaching the point when it is going to be necessary for us to work out something in line of a more close association."[26]

All this courting eventually paid off. Within a year west coast Canadians had grown weary of running a national organization without the help of, and often with the opposition of, easterners, while the easterners became more and more convinced that affiliation with an "efficiently functioning national organization" based on a large-scale membership was imperative." The ASA had such a membership base, the CSA did not. In July, 1953, Albert Taylor of Sunglades, now the newly elected national secretary of the CSA, met with "Pack" in Mays Landing, New Jersey, to discuss affiliation. They agreed in principle that the CSA could join the ASA and still retain its "national identity" and its own seat in the newly-formed International Naturist Federation (INF), which it joined in 1953. For Taylor affiliation was the best of both worlds: "the CSA would thus continue to have everything it now has, plus those things to be gained by being a part of the ASA."[27]

At the same 1954 convention that ratified CSA affiliation with the ASA, delegates rejected another pet project of their national secretary: renaming the CSA. Taylor argued that "sunbathing" was a "silly" term for a nudist organization and "nudist" was a term that people were "ashamed to mention in public," so he proposed "gymnosophical" as a substitute because no one "will know what it stands for" and therefore no nudist would have to worry about "ridicule or embarrassment." Gymnosophical was simple and straightforward: gymn(astics) plus (phil)osophical = gymnosophical. If this was not a more accurate description of nudism than sunbathing, it should be: "gymnastics, sports, games, or some other kind of physical activity . . . is absolutely essential, if one expects to derive the full benefit from nudism . . . . The Germans and the Swiss [Taylor was Swiss] certainly have the right spirit and seldom lie around in their camps."[28]

Taylor said the magic word. CSA officers rushed to defend the "democratic" right of Canadians to "lay in the sun and laze." Gymnastics might be all right for Germans—"it is part of their upbringing, they like being regimented"—but "we are democratic and we wish to be free." Besides, none of the "free and democratic" Canadians could spell or pronounce such a "foreign" word. Even Karl Ruehle, leader of Taylor's own club, pooh-poohed him: "he is too much stuck up with his vegetarian ideas, and his interest in better nutrition." Taylor defended his proposal in vain, for it became evident that this was an idea concocted in the east as a reaction against the western CSA for its past sins. Besides, Canadians did not see the point in changing the name of the Canadian Sunbathing Association at the same time as they affiliated with the American Sunbathing Association (unless Taylor proposed to convert Americans into "gymnosophists"). "We are a Canadian organization, so let us stick to a Canadian name."[29]

The 1955 convention set the stage and positioned the actors for the drama that would destroy the CSA. Ray Connett became National Secretary with a "salary" of one dollar per CSA member which he used to pay his typist. For the sake of this dollar Karl Ruehle, CSA Eastern Secretary with no salary, set out to break Connett, *Sunny Trails*, and the CSA. "The history of Canadian nudism is very much a story of the running battle between Karl Ruehle in the East and Ray Connett in the West."[30]

At first, Ray and Karl got along quite well. Ruehle actively and aggressively promoted his club, Sun Valley Gardens, and Connett—always a firm believer in publicity—congratulated him in September "on the splendid newspaper article you forwarded to me. It was a masterpiece, and I certainly admire the wonderful progress you have made in so short a time." And a little later, Ray offered Karl "the highest commendation" for his first press release.

"It was done up in a very sensible style and contained good sub-ject matter. Your first attempt was really an excellent one." For his part Karl appreciated the flattery and professed his willingness to learn from the master. "I must say that I am in this kind of dealing with the public still a poor orphan and are always ready to steal something from your vast experience."[31]

But when it came to Ruehle's role as eastern secretary for the CSA, Connett as national secretary was a more exacting taskmas-ter. When Karl cautioned Ontario nudists to be wary of an attempt to start a new indoor club in Toronto, Ray admonished him. "Really, Karl, I think this is uncalled for." This was the turning point in their relationship. From then on each man became more inflexible towards the other on a variety of issues, which separate-ly could have been resolved easily but which together reinforced their inflexible positions.[32]

By the spring of 1956 Karl and other Easterners were ready to declare war on Vancouver. "The national convention . . . will, can and must bring a change in CSA policies or a split between east and west might be possible." Ruehle wanted out from under Connett's control. He proposed a system whereby the national organization would "adopt all the aims of naturism" but would delegate substantive matters to the regionals to handle "suitable to their own preferred aims and taste . . . . The National body has no right to boss regionals but coordinates the main trend."[33]

The East botched every convention it held since 1948, and 1956 was no exception. The national convention was scheduled for a month before the regional convention in Vancouver, and the east sent the minutes of the national convention to the western region-al convention at "the slow cheap postage rate" instead of by air as requested, which forced the west to hold two conventions, with all the expense and inconvenience entailed.[34]

At the national convention, held at his own club, Karl Ruehle set out methodically to destroy the "Connett-controlled CSA." First, the east voted to break up the CSA—itself a regional association of the ASA—into three subregional organizations, each with its own executive board of five officers. The western convention modified this scheme to create an eastern and a western regional since there wasn't anyone inbetween. Each regional board would name three of its five members to a joint national board. The national president would be designated by each region in alternate years. Second, the east, becoming obsessed with cozy little family clubs, tried to disenfranchise all the CSA single members by restricting voting to club members and by denying singles the right to visit established clubs. The west defeated that proposal, and one that would have allowed proxy voting by clubs. Finally, the east tried to kill off Connett's *Sunny Trails* as the official CSA publication, and the west defeated that move also, on the grounds that there was no alternative available. But they did agree to an editorial review of the magazine.[35]

The east was not about to let a little thing like majority rule interfere with its concept of democracy. Although the west had vetoed two out of three eastern proposals, the one they won was the one that mattered: the east was now an autonomous division and from now on would be able to run its own divisional affairs without regard to western votes (except on constitutional matters). More important, Karl Ruehle was the new national secretary of the CSA despite the misgivings of Ray Connett and Marcus Meed, and his wife, Marlies, was secretary of the eastern division. It was time to make some changes.

After the 1956 convention, when the East overhauled the CSA without proposing constitutional amendments to accommodate these changes, the west accepted the eastern changes and set up a constitutional committee under Roy McKague, the first CSA president, to draft amendments that would reflect all changes made since 1947, including the 1954 merger with the ASA. This draft was circulated to Karl Ruehle, Marcus Meed, and Ray Connett before going to the two divisional conventions in 1957. The west accepted it (after a "good-natured laugh" about Karl and Marlies' newborn son making for a "new Ruehle" at Sun Valley Gardens) as delegates approved constitutional amendments reflecting the new structure. But once again the east refused to act in concert with the west and accepted only some of the changes while deleting and ignoring others and refusing to present alternative amendments.[36]

At the 1956 convention the east had voted to rescind the official status of *Sunny Trails* magazine but had been overruled by the west. At the divisional convention in 1957 the east did reject *Sunny Trails* (on a motion from Karl Ruehle) and voted to create its own magazine for club members, for CSA members, and for the general public. Karl Ruehle was "appointed or elected" editor and promptly announced that "I have taken over the job of getting the ball rolling." The untitled magazine "will not be a picture magazine but rather an interesting booklet with colorful contents, dealing with Naturism and Nudism, Art and History, Science and Culture, Biology and Medicine, and many other interesting items."[37]

As publisher of this encyclopedia Ruehle put the cart before the horse by attempting to line up paid subscriptions before anyone had a clear idea of what the magazine would look like. In August he invited "cooperation" but stressed the need for paid subscriptions first. A week later, in a letter to club owners and managers, Ruehle encouraged them to badger their members personally to subscribe. "I am sure no-one will be the one or few who are standing back and make themselves look cheap." He also threatened to send out his own reminders to all members who failed to subscribe.[38]

By this time clubs were growing restless under Ruehle's constant prodding. The Toronto club objected to the name of the magazine—*Canadian Naturist*—although Ruehle claimed that it had been selected "in democratic procedure" by the eastern division board. When the Toronto members hesitated to buy a new product sight unseen Ruehle suggested that the club should "instruct their members" what to do. TGS did not take kindly to criticism even when it did not come from Vancouver, and the club secretary complained to the eastern president in October that "many members spoke resentfully about the 'high pressure' nature of the propaganda for the Magazine." Although TGS recognized that the eastern convention had authorized the magazine and had appointed Ruehle as editor, "it was suggested that more courtesy would gain more support." Toronto also suggested that Ruehle was getting carried away in his ambitions for "a pretentious printed magazine" for public sale which would promote Ruehle's views on naturism. What Toronto wanted was a simple little newsletter reporting CSA news (something like *Sunny Trails*, perhaps?). Other clubs shared these sentiments, so when the executive board voted to review the magazine project Ruehle quit rather than submit to committee control, and the board voted to refund all subscription monies to members.[39]

Ruehle also found himself in trouble with Ed, the new president of the CSA East. During his term in office Ed split the east by his petty reaction to a petty expense deduction made by Ruehle after Karl and Marlies resigned from CSA office. When Ed refused to reimburse the "two or three dollars," Ruehle withheld all ASA/CSA membership fees until the next convention, when he paid in full except for himself and his wife. Ed used that as an excuse to read all members of Sun Valley out of the CSA, but this action was overruled, and the convention proceeded as usual. Along the way Ed generously invited Sun Valley members to join his London club, and this poisoned relations with Karl even further. "This man is through for me and a life time."[40]

But Ed was not through with Karl. The whole year after the 1958 convention was taken up with the "sordid personality conflict" between Karl and Ed and his wife, Jean, who replaced Marlies as eastern secretary. Although Jean admitted that "maybe Ed or the executive did make a mistake last year," they both refused to apologize to Karl and set out to make or break his club. "Karl has just got to learn that he is going to run his camp according to the C.S.A.A.S.A. rules and not Karl's." Ed and Jean rejected a suggestion from the national president that the CSA should cover Ruehle's currency exchange expenses since his was the only club with a large American membership. They invoked ASA by-laws, which stated that "all members of the local club shall be members of the Association and of the appropriate Regional Division" to counter Ruehle's claim that enough of his members were CSA/ASA to meet the minimum criteria for an ASA charter (ten adults), so that the rest of his 100+ membership need not join.[41]

The eastern division also quarrelled with its perennial nemesis, Ray Connett. The Toronto club tried to sort out eastern differences with him in a constructive manner. The TGS secretary shared eastern resentment over Connett's personal misuse of the official magazine: "it grieves me to see the CSA's official organ used for threshing out differences of opinion between various functionaries of the association." But Bill was more concerned over the inability of *Sunny Trails/Canadian Sun Air* to fulfill its constitutional function of publishing motions before the annual conventions to inform the membership. He blamed this failure on the magazine's irregular production schedule, which was caused in part by the problems associated with a one-man operation and in part by post office resistance to the nude pictures. TGS, like other clubs, refused to send pictures to Connett because "with every sympathy for lonely single men in northern construction camps, separated persons, etc., we didn't see why we should send our wives' and daughters' nude photos for them to lecher over." Bill proposed to address these problems by amending the constitution at the 1958 conventions.[42]

Throughout its history the "official organ" was plagued by problems which prevented it from fulfilling its mission. Some were technical problems with printers. In an attempt to control costs Connett searched far and wide for cheaper rates. For awhile the magazine was printed in Maple Creek, Saskatchewan, until the printer decided to move to Vancouver, which resulted in a delay of several issues. Later it was printed in India. Assistant editors came and went, format changed from mimeo to type to print and back, and the CSA, with a sigh of relief, returned the ownership to Ray and Mildred in 1950.[43]

The principal obstacle to publishing *Sunny Trails* on a regular basis was Post Office objection to the pictures. Connett believed a picture was worth a thousand words, and that pictures would show nudists in one club what nudists in other clubs were doing, and at the same time would prove to novices that nudists really were nude. Since the commercially distributed *Sunbathing for Health* seldom featured Canadian pictures, *Sunny Trails* was the only magazine providing pictorial evidence of Canadian nudism. But because *Sunny Trails* was mailed to CSA members and subscribers, it was subject to postal interference.

Starting in 1949 the Vancouver Post Office delayed release of the pre-convention issue because of pictures pending clarification from Ottawa, which authorized the mailing of that issue. In 1952 the Post Office struck again and banned the November issue, while the U.S. Postal Department imposed a ban against the CSA and its publications that remained in place until 1965. Connett believed that both actions were inspired by "that man in Montreal."[44]

When Connett wrote to the Investigations Division in Ottawa to protest the decision, noting that *Sunny Trails* was the official newsletter of the CSA, and requested postal guidelines on acceptable pictures, the answer was not very helpful: "pictures of nudist activities in which the human parts of the body are uncovered" were *verboten*. But Ottawa did agree to permit the November issue to be mailed without pictures. Connett reluctantly accepted this concession.[45]

Sunny Trails resumed publication in May, 1953, and continued for about a year before the next interruption, also caused by pictures. In January Connett had promised not to "use the mails in future for pictures of any nature disapproved of by the Department," and this gave him the opportunity to up the ante by offering to clear publication of pictures with local postal authorities. This worked on a temporary basis, but by spring of 1954 the Post Office tired of the game and again threatened to cut off mailing privileges for *Sunny Trails*. This resulted in another hiatus, from August 1954 to May 1955, when Connett again bowed to pressure.[46]

Postal threats were a two-fold danger for Connett. Not only did they disrupt publication of the official magazine of the CSA, but they jeopardized his own job as an employee of the post office. Ray was aware from the beginning that his high profile leadership position in the CSA might not ingratiate him with his supervisors, but decided that "a future of fear and uncertainty is a poor thing." But when the Post Office started banning *Sunny Trails* because of the "obscene" pictures they also warned him "that my job would be in jeopardy if I got in trouble with the magazine." He was demoted soon afterwards because his supervisors believed he was "more interested in my outside activities." It was for this reason that when the CSA returned ownership of the magazine to the Connetts in 1950 Mildred was listed as "technical owner of it in case I would be criticized by the Post Office." It was for this reason also that Connett tried, unsuccessfully, to enlist various assistant editors over the years. And it was for this reason that in 1957 Connett quit his job and moved to California. "I knew they would never give me a promotion. Who wants a nudist supervisor?"[47]

Throughout 1958-59 these concerns over Connett's self-styled role as reporter extraordinaire and as editor in chief of the two Canadian nudist magazines merged into one unremitting hatred of "Ray Connett and the Connett-controlled CSA." Ray persisted in his attempts to ferret out news, even if that meant "barking" at the east. Eventually his barking backfired, as Jean, the Eastern Secretary, caught between a constant stream of letters from Connett "putting his two cents in everywhere" and the steadfast policy of the eastern board to "answer all the questions that the Eastern Division Executive think are your business," found herself sorely tempted to join President Hank in resigning. In this attitude Jean reflected the sentiments of other eastern officers who felt that their business was "none of his business," including Don, the eastern publicity director and ASA trustee, and a future co-conspirator in the eastern plot to secede from the CSA once and for all, who assured Jean that "I will fire a blast at Ray in your support—what the blankety-blank has it to do with Ray anyway?"[48]

By spring 1959 time was running out. At the pre-convention

meeting the board and the club executives agreed that "the clubs were quite capable of running their own business;" that there was too much redundancy in administration between the clubs, the CSA East, CSA National, and the ASA; that there was too much correspondence— especially over "personality squabbles"—and not enough discussion; and that the simplest remedy for these problems was to reduce the geographical size of the eastern region and to reduce its ties to outside regions and organizations. Once Ontario became the center of the universe all would be right with the world.[49]

Now that the conspirators knew what they wanted the result of the convention to be, nudging the "small number of persons present" into agreement with their preconceived plan went smoothly. Since President Hank chose this moment to resign, past president Ed chaired the convention, which met at Sunshine Ranch on the weekend of 11-12 July 1959. After the opening formalities, Ed stepped up the pace by drawing attention to "the difficulties of operating under the existing CSA-ASA arrangements, chiefly owing to distance between Eastern and Western Clubs and other barriers to communication." Other delegates promptly chimed in with observations and proposals to support the federation idea. But the discussion of "the existing ASA arrangements" became heated when many loyalists argued that Canadians owed support to the ASA for its legacy to Canadian nudism, including its support during the Quetans trials, while opponents pointed not to the historic past but to the sordid present, in which "the ASA is riddled with internal dissention, clashes of personality, bickering over small issues, and bureaucratic procedures." The convention compromised on this issue by agreeing to seek a new "basis of affiliation," with less bureaucracy and lower cost. As for the CSA, no holds were barred.

> It was stated that Club Members resent the rule of officials who do not represent their Clubs, and who have been elected or appointed by Conventions which only a fraction of the Membership can attend. It was stated that CSA had been spoiled by squabbling and by publication of squabbling. A feeling was expressed that trouble results from appointing or electing people

to mind other people's business; that Clubs should run their own business, and be represented in all business concerning them.[50]

On Sunday, 12 July, Bill of TGS proposed that the CSA clubs in Ontario form a federation whose executive board would consist of the presidents of those clubs and who in turn would elect the chair from their ranks and that the federation would negotiate revised bases of affiliation with the CSA and the ASA. The delegates approved this plan by a vote of sixty-seven to one. Then, before anyone could have second thoughts, it was moved that the club presidents meet immediately to elect the new chair of the new board. After an afternoon of "good fellowship," the club presidents gathered to elect Chairman Ed, to christen their new organization the Ontario Federation of Nudist Clubs (OFNC), and to appropriate all CSA East money, including contributions from clubs that were now excluded from OFNC.[51]

The July convention set up OFNC as a federation of clubs. The routine correspondence would be handled by the one-man president/secretary/treasurer, Chairman Ed, and "major issues" would be referred to the club presidents for executive decision in a sort of board meeting by mail. This rather loose arrangement is what Chairman Ed meant when he informed the CSA that "we have fully set up our organization." He now proceeded to demonstrate what one vengeful but incompetent administrator could do if left unchecked. OFNC claimed to be the legal successor to the CSA eastern division (even though they wrote off all clubs east of Ontario), with full rights to all CSA eastern club members (in Ontario) and monies (from everywhere). Moreover, OFNC severed ties not only with the CSA but also with the ASA. Members who submitted renewal fees for ASA membership were issued OFNC cards instead. As Chairman Ed explained, "WE are not going to be a regional of ASA."[52]

These two actions—confiscation of CSA funds and secession from the ASA—"stopped the headlong progress of OFNC." When the handful of delegates at the convention got home they found their fellow club members—shocked and surprised at the action taken by the convention—demanding a new convention to reassess the July proceedings. In mid-August a "rally" of Toronto and Niagara members met at Sun Valley Gardens. This gathering declared that: (1) the CSA East "is still in existence," even though the 1959 convention failed to elect any officers; members of CSA and ASA remained members of these organizations; clubs remain affiliated with ASA unless and until OFNC negotiated new terms for affiliation (but not membership: the East wanted to belong to the ASA for fifty cents per year instead of four dollars); eastern division funds remained the property of the CSA until a proper and legal transition from CSA eastern division to OFNC occurred. Each and every one of these four points repudiated the official line of Chairman Ed—that OFNC was the legal successor to the CSA East because it had been created at a convention that was supposed to be a CSA convention.[53]

By this time the CSA national board had entered the fray. In late July 1959 Chairman Ed forwarded a copy of the convention minutes to Vancouver, along with a letter stating that, since the convention created a new organization, the East "will not have any officers as far as CSA National Board [is] concerned." The CSA responded with mixed feelings. In principle, Ray Connett felt that OFNC was "an excellent idea," but regretted the haste with which the motion was pushed through without any regard for constitutional niceties. "No one who has worked long and hard for Canadian nudism can view current events without a trace of sadness. The thought of a divided Canada is repugnant to any Canadian."[54]

Soon the west began receiving letters from the east that led them to realize that not everyone was sold on the OFNC idea. Thus the CSA national board felt obliged to act on behalf of those CSA East members who opposed OFNC. The ASA authorized the CSA president to appoint replacements for the eastern officers not elected by the eastern convention. In mid-September the CSA decided to demand that Ed provide the national office with a financial report on CSA East funds, since there had been no report at the July convention. Not trusting Ed to comply with this request, the CSA president also wrote to past officers of the CSA East to ask for their assistance. "The minutes do not show any motion authorizing a transfer or any disposition of CSA-E funds. Therefore, we can only conclude that if these funds have been transferred into an account under the name of O.F.N.C. it has not been a legal action."[55]

After a month of further correspondence Ed agreed to deposit the pro-rata share of CSA East funds in a separate CSA East account for all clubs "not authorizing transfer to OFNC." There still remained the question of all CSA records, correspondence, and other property which "you hold without any valid legal, moral, or even ethical excuse." These issues would not be resolved until a joint East-West committee was set up in January to divide all CSA materials.[56]

In its haste to undo everything the west had accomplished in the CSA, the east tried persistently to destroy affiliation with the ASA, even though the east had imposed that affiliation on the west in 1954. At the July convention "considerable discussion ensued as to the advisability or otherwise of the proposed federation being completely independent of the American Sunbathing Association." The convention authorized the federation to "nego- tiate a revised basis of affiliation" with the ASA.[57]

This set the stage for another round of confusion as Ed acted one way and the clubs another. In mid-August, when Ed was informing Ray Connett bluntly that "WE are not going to be a regional of ASA," the Ontario clubs wrote a collective letter to Ed stating that "we are still members of the ASA" and demanding that "C.S.A.-A.S.A. cards must still be obtained." East Haven, the Maritans, Niagara, Norhaven, Sunny Brae, and Toronto all made it clear that "affiliation with the A.S.A. is a must." To all these con- cerns Chairman Ed replied obstinately that when the OFNC was formed the "CSA Eastern Division ceased to be. OFNC cards will be issued as ASA cards come up for renewal." This prompted the Toronto club, one of the principal supporters of OFNC, to caution

Ed about his handling of the affiliation issue: "a good deal of thought should go into any correspondence."[58]

By this time it was becoming clear that OFNC would remain with the ASA. Throughout the autumn, as opposition to OFNC mounted within Ontario, the CSA held open the possibility of separate regional status for OFNC. Chairman Ed remained the chief obstacle to this felicitous reconciliation. He thwarted CSA efforts to obtain eastern CSA/ASA records in order to assist those clubs that preferred ASA affiliation over OFNC and dragged his feet when most of the OFNC clubs accepted the ASA proposal for a summit conference in January to resolve the whole OFNC mess. While everyone else started to prepare for the meeting Ed wrote to the ASA in December that "OFNC does not intend to be a Regional of the ASA, " and he explained his reasons to one of his active collaborators in Toronto, who happened to be the ASA trustee for the CSA East. "I am standing behind the OFNC idea of being a separate organization and not a Regional of ASA." Provincial FNCs would still mean "ASA tons of red tape" which OFNC (and Ed in particular) wanted to escape. For his part Don, the ASA Trustee, was equally oblique in dealing with Vancouver, telling Ray Connett that OFNC "did NOT decide to leave ASA or CSA," while assuring Ed that "our relationship with ASA must be set up so that we bypass CSA national, but don't let Pack or CSA National realize this until agreement is reached."[59]

By December it was clear that "OFNC did not immediately pan out as the New Heaven and the New Earth for the nudist movement in Ontario." As Marcus Meed, one of OFNC's orphans, put it, "the present situation in the East would be comical if it were not so pathetic." In order to resolve the "bloody mess" and put OFNC back on track, TGS called on Chairman Ed to provide copies of all OFNC correspondence since July. When it received this correspondence and saw how many different things Ed had been telling different people they finally understood why all the other clubs opposed them.[60]

In January 1960 the CSA National and the ASA convened a

joint CSA/OFNC/ASA meeting to sort out the mess in Ontario. On the weekend of 23-24 January fifteen representatives from OFNC clubs—half of them from the London Sun Club in support of Chairman Ed—gathered at the Royal York Hotel in Toronto to meet with Norval Packwood, executive director of the ASA, to "explore all angles of the matter of the ASA, the CSA, and the OFNC, in the hope of reaching a basis for understanding." After twenty-five hours of discussion, "laying our cards on the table," the delegates reached a consensus calling for the re-creation of the CSA Eastern Division on the basis of OFNC rules of procedure, the separation of the east from the west in two autonomous regionals of the ASA, and the relegation of the CSA to "a fellowship of Canadian Nudist Clubs, but without administrative functions."[61]

After eastern clubs had the chance to consider the report of the January meeting the secretary of TGS drafted a constitution for the reconstructed regional association. The new constitution would perpetuate the spirit of OFNC in a more "democratic" framework, provide for affiliation with the ASA, and "prevent the domination of eastern Canadian nudism through the *Canadian Sun Air* magazine."

> From this it seems to me that all the ritual of forming a new Regional can quite happily drag out until kingdom come. Meanwhile, we can pay our ASA $4 and get protection and benefits accordingly; we can have our OFNC conventions for fun and games, include and indoctrinate the new and the dissident clubs, and take any formal notes required in the tortuous processes of ASA law; nobody on earth can force us to pay a cent or send a name to CSA.[62]

The new constitution was discussed and accepted at the first of two eastern conventions during the summer of 1960. In June, club representatives gathered at Glen Echo to undo the damage caused by the 1959 convention (Chairman Ed did not attend). Acknowledging that the previous convention had not abolished the CSA eastern division but had merely sabotaged it, Bill proposed that the eastern division and the western division apply to the CSA and the ASA for ASA status as independent regional associations, and that they negotiate an equitable division of all CSA records and funds.[63]

In August 1960 the ASA national convention approved unanimously the formation of the two Canadian regionals—the ECSA and the WCSA. Ray Connett had written earlier that "this can easily mean the beginning of a remarkable new era of progress in Canadian nudism," and his eastern critics replied in kind.

> We have fought and feuded with him, we have disagreed with him and complained most bitterly about him but we all know that his enthusiasm and constant needling has kept us all on our toes and spurred us on to do those things we have done. It is only fitting that this portion of the history of the development of nudism should close with the name of the grand-father of it all—Ray Connett.[64]

CHAPTER ELEVEN

The Three Solitudes

After four years of struggle the east was free at last. But its independence was not unfettered. Just as the first secession in 1956 remained incomplete, so too 1960 represented only a partial victory. The east had indeed destroyed the CSA, but at the price of continued affiliation with the ASA. And nothing had been done to silence Ray Connett, whose *Canadian Sun Air* remained the official publication of the WCSA and, implicitly, of the residual CSA, which still existed in however disembodied a form—another concession that the OFNC conspirators had been forced to grant. These constraints set the ECSA agenda for the next four years: to break Ray Connett once and for all and to quit the ASA at the earliest opportunity.

At the August 1960 convention at the London Sun Club, delegates endorsed the draft constitution which established the Eastern Canadian Sunbathing Association as the proper successor to the CSA East. Members of each club would elect a delegate to represent them on the ECSA board, which would conduct business by correspondence and report to the members for approval and for voting whenever necessary. All in all, the constitution was presented as a "masterpiece of simplicity." The ECSA set out to show the nudist world how democracy works.[1]

The first step for the new organization was to put its erstwhile enemies in their place. Karl Ruehle was already out, on his own initiative, and with no regrets. Ruehle and the ECSA maintained an ambivalent relationship over the years. The association welcomed Sun Valley members as guests to conventions but refused to invite Karl himself. Karl naturally reciprocated these sentiments, regarding the ECSA as "sneaky" and untrustworthy.

> If you can take a well-meant advise from someone
> who knows all the people who are now running the
> ECSA, then watch out and trust not those who are so
> very diplomatic but cut you short where ever they
> can, and you don't notice where it comes from.[2]

The war of words between Ray Connett and the east continued after 1960. Because of his stature as the elder statesman of the movement, many people not actively involved in the new organization still looked to Connett for advice and assistance, even though he no longer held any Canadian position and resided in California. When internal trouble disrupted the East Haven club in 1960 and the two protagonists contacted Connett, he immediately advised both to deal with the ECSA. For its part the ECSA ignored this gesture of cooperation and cautioned the disputants against writing to Connett. And when Connett tried to stir up discussion of the ECSA's "new form of government" in the July 1961 issue of *Sun Air* the ECSA refused to fall into the baited trap. Dissatisfaction lingered even in the west, and Connett became increasingly discouraged by the dwindling number of subscribers and by the WCSA's decision to revoke its "official publication" status. In the April 1964 issue (released in August) Connett announced "the end of Canadian Sun Air, which has brought you news and views of Canadian nudist activity since 1947."[3]

With the disappearance of *Sun Air* the two Canadian regions became responsible for their own publications. The WCSA launched its own *Newsletter*, later renamed *Canadian Nudist News*. The ECSA had rejected *Sun Air* in 1960 and started producing the ECSA Newsletter to provide "AUTHENTIC news. Nothing from other sources shall be taken as official." In 1965 the ECSA published the *Sunshine Family*, a guide to all ECSA clubs, featuring information and pictures (mainly from the Toronto and London clubs) and intended for public distribution "to attract the responsible families of Canada."[4]

Having disposed of its Canadian opponents, the ECSA set out to eliminate the American connection. It would enter the ASA in order to demonstrate how democracy works. If the ASA learned from the ECSA model and reformed itself, the ECSA might remain affiliated. If not, then the OFNC, "which is dormant but not dead," offered an alternative. "Unless and until ASA improves greatly, we can expect the question of our secession from it to come up from time to time."[5]

The first opportunity for the pupil to instruct the teacher occurred at the moment of birth for the ECSA region. As a responsible Regional of the ASA, the ECSA felt obliged to submit a resolution to the parent organization calling on "ASA authorities to direct their energies once again to the promotion of the democratic processes by which disputes can be resolved and the greater goals attained." These "democratic processes" involved the reorganization of the ASA so that all business would be conducted by regional trustees through correspondence, with conventions limited to "fun, fellowship, and sport," with "no governing powers." The ECSA assumed, perversely, that all national associations were the creations of the regional associations, when in fact the opposite was true—it was the national associations that spawned the regional associations in both countries. But the real reasons for the ECSA's opposition to "convention government" were the inability of the CSA East to get its own way within the national CSA and the provincial easterners' inability or unwillingness to attend conventions outside Ontario.[6]

The first warning that all was not well came when the ECSA learned that its proposals had not been placed before the national convention but sent to committee—"the proverbial trash basket." In April 1962 the ECSA reintroduced a resolution that the next ASA convention agree in principle to amend the by-laws to designate the board of trustees as the general governing body, responsible to the club members of the regional associations, instead of acting like "an unwelcome senior Aunt bossing the family of Regions around in a pointless parlor-game." It was now that the ECSA felt in full force the "dictatorial manner" of the ASA president, Sol Stern, when he unilaterally voided the ECSA's resolution and instructed the ECSA on the proper procedure for submitting proposals to the ASA. "If this is a manifestation of your understanding of the doctrine of chain of command, it explains the cause of many of the problems that have plagued your Regional."[7]

Since its attempt to follow standard procedure had been thwarted by the ASA president, the ECSA decided to swallow its pride and do what sympathizers had long advised them to do: send a delegate to the ASA convention to make sure that its voice was heard. At the ASA convention everything—as usual—was tabled. This was done in part because delegates agreed with the ECSA in principle but did not want to rock the boat at an otherwise "harmonious" convention, in part because Stern was no longer president, and in part because it was lunch time and no one wanted to debate anything. At least the ECSA could take consolation in the fact that the ASA convention named Ray Connett the official "Court Jester."[8]

By the summer of 1963 the situation in the ASA was "obviously getting worse, and showing no sign of ability to improve." The ECSA proposals on restructuring the ASA were referred back to committee for the third straight year; the chair of the finance committee quit because he "felt he was not needed;" and the ASA proposed a new constitution, which, instead of fostering more democracy in the ECSA manner, would "wipe out the Regionals and seize their funds." Under the circumstances the ECSA convention authorized the board to "initiate Constitution Amendments to delete reference to A.S.A."[9]

Board members had been waiting for this moment since 1960. In January 1964 club members cast their votes "overwhelmingly in favor of independence"—three-fourths of all club members voted on the ballot, ninety per cent in favor of separation—and on 15 February 1964 the ECSA officially left the ASA. ASA national headquarters responded bluntly, writing off the puny four hundred member regional, its inconsequential financial contribution of less than $1,000 per year, and its insignificant contribution to the political life of the ASA.[10]

On all counts the ECSA failed miserably after 1964. It barely scraped together membership dues for the INF and never placed a Canadian on the INF board; the only large-scale publicity project in Canada during the 1960s and 1970s was the Miss Nude World contest organized by the Four Seasons club; the only representation the ECSA ever made to government was to write a letter to thank Leo Bernier, Ontario Minister of Natural Resources, after he suggested that provincial parks ought to accommodate a wider variety of public groups, possibly including nudists; and the only pressures on magazine publishers were negative—the ECSA helped destroy *Sunbathing for Health* and *Canadian Sun Air*—or futile, since the American and European magazine publishers did not concern themselves with the views of a pipsqueak organization that eventually represented only one hundred members.[11]

What proved truly fatal for the ECSA was its inability to mobilize and satisfy the several hundred members that it had inherited from the CSA. The more that members withdrew into their shells, the less they wanted to visit other clubs or to be visited by other nudists, especially if they had to pay for the privilege at convention time. In 1969 the ECSA restructured fees so that "services will be paid for by those who demand them and use them." Everyone who wanted nothing paid one dollar per year; special events were to be self-supporting.[12]

These changes led the board to draft a series of amendments to the constitution that would incorporate a statement of beliefs, standards, and purposes to replace the ASA guidelines, reduce fees to a bare-bones level of one dollar per family per year, and allow club owners as well as members to represent their clubs on the board. The ECSA circulated these amendments to its clubs in the spring of 1971 for a June vote. After a majority of "those few members" who voted in June opposed the amendments, several of the larger clubs, including Glen Echo, Ponderosa, and Sunny Glades, severed ties with the organization. This created a new problem for the ECSA—marshalling a quorum for board meetings—since the clubs that remained affiliated were small and widely scattered (e.g. Bel Air and SilvaSun in eastern Ontario and Temiskaming Heliosophical Society in northern Ontario). To solve this problem

President Jim convened a board meeting in 1972 to "expel or suspend the three remaining clubs" so that the board could coast on a quorum of two representatives thereafter. This was admittedly a desperate expedient, but, as the president noted to another board member and ECSA founding father, "I seem to be stalemated and hanged by the constitution!"[13]

He was also stalemated by apathy on the board, encountering a complete "absence of any form of leadership from our officers." A special meeting was convened on 6 May 1972 to elect new officers, expel old clubs, hold on to the remaining little clubs, and consider the future. On one point the ECSA board and the disillusioned dropout clubs agreed: they were all hoist by the constitutional petard.[14]

In August the board decided once again to amend the constitution. Perhaps with most of the 1971 members gone, the small remainder might approve the revisions. The principal innovations included board representation of both owners and members (rather than requiring owners to be elected in order to represent their own club), extending the geographical scope of the ECSA to embrace all of Canada (since Ontario was a washout), and removing the age-old ASA rules against alcohol and common-law marriages. To ensure safe passage, the board claimed that since this was a new constitution rather than an amendment to the existing one, the constitutional provision regarding amendments "is not applicable." Four clubs approved the changes, two did not reply ("abstaining by default"), and so the board decided that the ECSA had a new constitution after all.[15]

Having changed its constitution, its domain, and its behavior, the ECSA decided to change its name as well; at the 1973 convention the ECSA became the Canadian Nudist Confederation (CNC). "We feel that the new name adopted at our Executive Meeting and Convention in August 1973 is in greater keeping with our Nationalistic outlook and reflects the contributions of our French speaking members." The francophone members came from Bel Air, site of the 1973 convention; the "nationalistic outlook" came from two western additions to the ranks of CNC in 1974: the Van Tans and the Canadian Sun Ranch Association.[16]

Downsizing came with a price—$2,000, divided among all the ECSA clubs when the largest clubs left or were asked to leave after the 1971 convention. Most of the disbursement came from the defense fund which seemed to have no purpose in a Canada without Maurice Duplessis, "so why finance a legal fund that would never be used." After the 1972 restructuring the ECSA/CNC was left with assets of $130, or about one dollar per member—and the board offered most of that reserve to the WCSA as a bribe to forget the old 1960 references to preserving the CSA as "a fellowship of Canadian nudist clubs." Since this amount equalled the total of annual dues, the "limited finances" precluded giving out copies of the constitution to the remaining members. The ECSA/CNC was also unable to reclaim its convention games trophies from one of the dropout clubs: the owner did not think that the "little group" could do anything to get them back, and the board had to agree, since they couldn't afford a lawyer.[17]

After nearly a decade of limited accomplishment, activity, interest, and involvement, there came a time when board members had to decide "should C.N.C. continue?" On April Fools' Day, 1978, the board members recorded the verdict they had all reached independently over the years and voted to dissolve the CNC once and for all.[18]

The events of 1959-1960 naturally affected Western Canadians. In late June 1960 the CSA West met in convention at Sol Sante to adopt in principle a draft constitution defining the Western Canadian Sunbathing Association (WCSA) as an independent regional of the ASA, requiring that all members of all affiliated clubs must be members of the WCSA/ASA, and inaugurating a new voting formula adopted in 1959 whereby club "delegates" rather than individual members would cast votes at conventions (although all members were welcome to attend and to participate in discussion). All clubs were entitled to two delegates for the first twenty-five members and one additional delegate for each additional twenty-five members. Officers would be elected for a two-year term, and had to have held club membership for at least two years.[19]

The 1961 convention at Sunny Trails (held for the first time in July, because after fourteen years members finally realized that it rains during June in British Columbia), members voted to accept the constitution proposed in 1960, but with one issue unresolved: club representation on the board. The WCSA opted to conduct a mail ballot on this issue among club delegates from the 1961 convention after those delegates consulted with their home clubs. This allowed the constitution business to drag on for two more years, until the 1963 convention at Sol Sante, when it "was accepted with one amendment and is now in force." The WCSA also decided to incorporate under the Societies Act in order to function as a legal entity.[20]

For much of its history the WCSA (now WCANR) has agonized over the question of affiliation with the ASA. In what must have been a bitter disappointment for Ray Connett, now active in the Western Sunbathing Association in California, the first club to quit the WCSA was his own Sunny Trails Club, in 1962. The decision was all the more painful for all parties because Sunny Trails was slated to host the ASA convention that year. Bailing out on short notice started "the 'poor mouth' reputation of the Western Canadians" and provoked some Americans in 1964 to try and "squeeze us out of the A.S.A. because we only had three chartered clubs." This happened in the same year that the ECSA left the ASA, and it required heroic efforts by Ernie Detwiller, the only Canadian delegate at the ASA convention, to stave off this threat.[21]

Next to go was Sol Sante. This "little club" hosted the ASA convention in 1965 before it had developed the facilities to handle a national gathering (partly because it hoped to use the resulting income to pay for those facilities), and the "rustic" conditions as well as the distance kept many Americans away. Sol Sante left the WCSA/ASA in 1967.[22]

The Van Tan Club considered leaving the ASA as early as 1961.

In 1967 it passed a motion to "sever its affiliation and press for for-mation of a purely Canadian parent organization"—this in response to friendly correspondence with the ECSA, now outside the ASA. But discussion with WCSA representatives dissuaded the Van Tans temporarily. In 1971 the club did vote to leave the WCSA, and later it tried to establish contact with a more sympa-thetic CNC in the east. But when its eastern ally folded the Van Tans reappraised the joy of solitude and reaffiliated with the WCSA/ASA.[23]

The loss of two landed clubs in B.C. and the imminent prospect of losing more left the WCSA "wobbly" and forced it to reconsid-er its future. In 1968 the WCSA set up a Committee to Investigate the Pros and Cons of Affiliation. Then in the early 1970s a new wave of separatist sentiment struck. In spring of 1971 Sol Sante proposed formation of a Western Canadian Naturist Group (WCNG). To some clubs this looked worse than the ASA because of the provision for expulsion of members "with no right to due process, fair trial, or appeal." Given Sol Sante's own checkered history of internal purges the WCNG did not hold much appeal for other western clubs. None the less, Sol Sante staged a founding convention for the Western Canadian Naturist Group. They did not explain how this new group differed from the WCSA/ASA arrangement, except for its proposed dues of one dollar per member.[24]

At the 1971 convention the Van Tan Club, which had just voted to give one year's notice of disaffiliation, presented a motion "that the WCSA give one year's notice of its intent to disaffiliate on a friendly basis from the ASA at the 1972 WCSA convention." To the surprise of everyone the motion passed, and even though the ASA president tried to claim that the ASA owned its regionals and that the WCSA could not leave, his own ASA convention voted to allow regionals to disaffiliate at will. A new Dissolution Committee under a new chairman set out to find a formula that would allow "the rebels" to create "a new independent Canadian Nudist Organization" without prejudicing the right of individuals or clubs to remain affiliated with the ASA.[25]

In the autumn of 1971 the WCSA board rejected the committee's draft constitution for a Canadian Naturist Federation because it presumed a new name and a new direction for the association.

> Have you noticed the ASA Loyalists, who are fighting hard for a strong WCSA, are mainly Nudists born in Canada, while the majority of Rebels advocating a "Truly Canadian" organization were born Overseas? [26]

The ASA presidential assistant for WCSA affairs argued that foreigners had not lived in Canada long enough to understand the blind Canadian faith in everything American, yet he claimed that his one year in England qualified him to denounce categorically everything that British naturism represented. After the 1971 convention voted to give notice of intent to withdraw, Ron wrote an open letter to the WCSA president objecting to certain foreign influences corrupting the good judgment of real Canadians and undermining the WCSA's proper subservience to the ASA. [27]

In 1972 the Van Tan Club finally quit the WCSA. Although several new clubs formed in British Columbia and affiliated with the WCSA, all were small travel clubs, which could not compensate the association for the loss of the three largest landed clubs. In recognition of that fact, and the corresponding dearth of west coast officers, the WCSA's 1972 convention elected a new board, whose husband-and-wife-team of president and secretary were from Crocus Grove in Manitoba: "finally the responsibility for the conduct of the Western Canadian Sunbathing Association has passed east of the mountains." But the transfer was a mixed blessing, as the new president's "dictatorial habits" disturbed many seasoned officers who resented having reports tabled because of his "let's get out of here and have a party" attitude. The frat-house approach to business so disrupted WCSA affairs that the new president became an ex-president midway through his term, with the threat of legal action against him because of his continuing obstruction of association business. In 1973 the WCSA simplified the procedure for removing "negligent" officers. "We are going ahead and will not tolerate people who take a position for the title and then do little or nothing." [28]

This experience, along with the growing number of clubs (though not of members), prompted the WCSA to review its constitution once again. In 1972, after the convention defeated the motion to quit the ASA, Ernie Detwiller was appointed to chair a Legislation Committee to revise the constitution to streamline association business and to facilitate incorporation. After considering the option of incorporating in each of the western provinces, the WCSA decided to seek a federal charter. But this almost brought about disaffiliation by itself, for Canadian law would not allow ASA policy and procedure to take precedence over Canadian policy and procedure. Legally, the WCSA became a separate corporation on an equal level with its "parent" ASA, with which it could maintain only a "fraternal" affiliation. When the WCSA asked Ottawa, "is there any way possible that we can be a member of and not just affiliated fraternally with The American Sunbathing Association," the answer was a categorical "No." As their own solicitor explained, the WCSA was "an independent organization with only 'fraternal' affiliation with the American Sunbathing Association. Therefore, your constitution and bylaws are dominant and their constitution and bylaws have no legal effect whatsoever . . . The American Association bylaws would have a moral persuasiveness due to your fraternal affiliation but would not be legally binding on your Association."[29]

In 1983 the parent ASA changed its rule requiring 100 per cent membership and allowed clubs to choose their own terms for affiliation. The Van Tans took advantage of the offer and rejoined the ASA in 1985. But the very next year the WCSA once again discussed a proposal to quit the ASA. Then in 1993, recognizing the importance of nude recreation for the future, the ASA and the WCSA changed their name. After more than half a century as a sunbathing association, concerns about ozone and melanoma, as well as a belated recognition that more people are nudists outside clubs than inside, prompted the ASA to become the American Association for Nude Recreation (AANR). The WCSA led the way in adopting the new name: "That is what we do, we recreate in the nude." But no sooner had the WCSA converted to the WCANR than it criticized the parent/fraternal organization for trying to raise dues forty per cent (in effect) by requiring Canadians to pay in U.S. dollars. The WCANR defeated this proposal—as it had all previous such efforts—but the need constantly to fend off American depredations helped weaken those fraternal bonds. Not a few westerners realized that there were alternatives to "Big Brother," and some tried to revive the idea of the Western Canadian Naturist Association in case "we ever dare come together with our eastern fellow naturists." Helios Edmonton left AANR in 1998 and joined the Federation of Canadian Naturists, and since then most Western clubs have joined the FCN, while retaining affiliation with the WCANR/AANR.[30]

In a 1977 magazine article surveying the situation of nudism in Quebec, François Huot posed the rhetorical question, "When will there be a Quebec federation of naturism? When will there be cooperation between naturist clubs and the provincial federations of socio-cultural leisure activities and outdoor recreation?"[31] The answer came quickly, for at that very moment a group of individuals meeting at the Pommerie club decided to organize the Fédération Québécoise de Naturisme (FQN), or Quebec Federation of Naturism.

Michel Vaïs, founder of the FQN, had discovered naturism while in France for doctoral studies. After reading *La Vie au Soleil*, the glossy French nudist magazine, Vaïs decided to visit one of the oceanside clubs, Montalivet, and became hooked. He returned home in 1974 determined to continue the naturist lifestyle in Quebec. He found, to his pleasant surprise, that during his years away Quebec had experienced a virtual explosion of nudist clubs. But all these clubs were isolated endeavors with no interconnection or cooperation. The only bond that they had in common was the tabloid *Nudistes du Québec*, which most of them regarded as a "veritable smut rag." Moreover, the clubs operated only during the summer season; there were no year-round activities of the sort Vaïs came to appreciate while in France.[32]

Vaïs established contact with the clubs and their members, and in 1976, after reading about a club being started near Montreal, La

Pommerie, founded by Jean Marcel Boucher, whom Vaïs met at a resort in Corsica in 1974, he joined that club. Then, in spring 1977, when La Pommerie opened for its first season, Vaïs posted notices asking people interested in forming a Quebec organization to gather for a meeting there on 29 May. Throughout that summer there would be many such meetings, culminating in the granting of provincial letters patent to the *Féderation québécoise de naturisme* on Bastille Day, 14 July 1977. And in August the FQN set up several committees to prepare a constitution, by-laws, rules and regulations, and generally to define the scope of the organization.[33]

The situation facing the organizers was promising. Nudism already had a foothold in Quebec, with several well-established clubs and the biweekly tabloid *Nudistes du Québec*. But persuading the other players to accept the fledgling federation as the central coordinator proved difficult. Club owners were intensely suspicious, regarding their clubs as a private domain and their members as captive serfs. They objected to the FQN's self-styled role as coordinator of nudism in Quebec—"who are you to organize us?"—and to the FQN's emphasis on European style naturism which did not sit well with their more familiar North American style nudism: "Montreal is not Paris." Behind all these suspicions and objections lay an inability to believe that the FQN leaders "were crazy enough to work voluntarily for the development of naturism." For its part the FQN, in its bid to represent Quebec in the INF, denounced the Federation of Quebec Nudist Clubs to the INF for advertising in *Nudistes du Québec*.[34]

Jean Marc Provost, publisher of *Nudistes du Québec*, also regarded the FQN with suspicion. When the Federation contacted him in November 1977, "knowing your interest with respect to naturism and the active role which you play through your paper," and asked for a meeting to discuss "the best way to promote naturism in Quebec," he questioned the need for a "naturist" federation and its "naturist" objectives—"words! just words empty of meaning"—and implied that the federation would exist to make money for its organizers and to impose naturism on the clubs by banning beer, meat, and smoking.[35]

None of these initiatives succeeded in defining the *raison d'être* of the FQN. When members held their first general assembly on 24 February 1978, "it was hard to know how to begin." *Faute de mieux*, the FQN became an organization based on individual rather than on club membership. It would publicize naturism through the media, make representations to government, and promote alternative recreation activities for unorganized naturists at indoor sports facilities and free beach areas.[36]

In 1978, in connection with the preparation of a Green Book on sports and recreation by the new provincial government, the FQN submitted a brief calling for greater governmental acceptance of and support for naturism. The FQN made three specific recommendations: recognition of the right to nudity (i.e. decriminalization); creation of designated free beach areas; and access to public (municipal) recreational facilities for naturist recreation, such as municipal swimming pools).[37]

In the summer of 1979 the FQN applied to join the Confederation de Loisir du Quebec. The CLQ denied the application "for the time being" in order to give the FQN the opportunity to establish itself more securely within Quebec and to attain "a truly national dimension," at which time the Confederation would reconsider the request. In 1980 the FQN established its first regional chapter, in Quebec City, and continued its promotional activities. In the spring of 1981 it mounted a strong presentation at the Camping Show in Place Bonaventure.[38] These successful efforts prompted the CLQ—now renamed the Regroupement des Organismes Nationaux de Loisir du Quebec (RONLQ)—to invite the FQN to reapply for affiliation, which it did on April 10. One month later RONLQ accepted the FQN. After overcoming some procedural snags, the FQN moved into the offices of the Secretariat des Organismes de Loisir du Quebec (SOLQ—the administrative arm of RONLQ), and in 1985 they all took up new quarters in the Olympic Stadium, where the FQN remains.[39]

Affiliation with RONLQ was a major step for the FQN and "opened big doors for many services." The Regroupement, though an autonomous association of scores of recreational organizations, was subsidized by the Quebec government and was able to provide its affiliates with office space, equipment, and services, including support services for the production of brochures, newsletters, and magazines. It also lends an indefinable cachet of respectability to its affiliates that was especially valuable for a nudist organization. Unfortunately, the FQN was never able to parlay its membership in RONLQ into direct subsidy from the provincial government, which argued that naturism is not a recreational practice but an ensemble of recreational practices such as swimming and volleyball. Since the government did subsidize other "ensemble" organizations, the FQN naturally concluded that "the decision whether to subsidize naturists is a political one."[40]

In June 1979 the FQN issued its first *Bulletin d'Information*, which became *Les Informations naturistes québécoises*. From the very beginning the Federation was anxious to avoid identification with *Nudistes du Québec*. It chose articles and pictures to reflect the philosophy and practice of naturism. The bulletin was directed not only to members but to the general public and was sold in newsstands. After the FQN joined RONLQ it was able to produce a more professional-looking magazine and in 1982 decided to rename its publication in an open contest. Although in hindsight the final choice—*Au Naturel*—appears obvious, members submitted nearly fifty names, most of them containing variations on nude, nature, and sun. The final choice appeared on Issue 12: *Au Naturel*. The magazine reported on FQN organization activities, club life, free beaches, naturism, and natural health topics. Although RONLQ provided technical services to assist in production, the FQN had to cover most of the costs, and, given its limited finances, the magazine ran a deficit every year. Starting in the mid-1980s the board intermittently dropped issues and substituted "newsletters" and "bulletins" in an effort to economize, but to no avail. The deficit continued to climb, despite generous donations from members and fundraising ventures such as selling Lotto tickets and staging auctions. In the 1990s the magazine appeared sporadically, and in 2000 not at all. At that time the FQN reverted to the original format and produced a newsletter, *Le Lien Naturiste*.

To take up the slack, the founding president started a new magazine, *Naturisme Québec.*[41]

In addition to its publications, the FQN adopted a forthright publicity campaign. From the outset it gave notices of events such as winter swims to newspapers. FQN representatives gave interviews to the press, radio, and television. On one notable occasion (3 May 1985), twenty nudists—half from the FQN, the others from clubs and beaches—appeared on a Radio Québec tv program "Droit de parole aux nudistes," hosted by Claire Lamarche. Although advance publicity by the network suggested titillation— "Are they voyeurs? Are they exhibitionists? Or, people concerned with their health?"—the program itself gave a balanced presentation of the nudist philosophy and nudist experience. A number of the estimated 400,000 viewers called the network to congratulate it and the FQN: "it's about time that someone spoke about this virtually unexplored subject." But others were less content, calling the show "stupid," "vulgar," and "decadent" because "it's not very good for the kids" and suggesting that the government should abolish the network for showing the program.[42]

Special interest exhibitions are another publicity forum for the FQN. Some of the Quebec clubs had participated on their own in events like the Montreal Camping Show, but in 1981 the FQN "took a great step forward" by entering its own display booth at the show, in Place Bonaventure. Forty members staffed the booth and offered to "discuss the question of naturism with the general public for the first time." They distributed club brochures, FQN bulletins, and 5,000 copies of the glossy *Vie au Soleil*. As the FQN president reported, "the camping show has been incontestedly the chief engine of our publicity campaign this year." In later years the FQN placed a booth at camping shows, sportsman shows, vacation shows, and youth Shows. The booth displayed posters and literature, and screened ASA and FQN nudist videos on tv monitors.[43]

FQN relations with clubs remained ambivalent. Some owners, impressed with its publicity work at the exhibitions and in the media, joined the Federation on an individual basis, and two even served on the board. In return the FQN adopted the term "friendly clubs" and printed news of their activities in *Au Naturel*. In 1983 the FQN offered "a specific package of services" for club membership. It provided a level of promotion and publicity that was beyond the reach of the clubs separately, in return for an open house day for FQN members with free admission and no quotas— something that they called "a simple matter of justice." The FQN also called on its "accredited clubs" to provide "a recreational setting as much as possible compatible with the naturist ideal (exclusion or control of ordinary nuisances: noise, pollution, commercial promotions, sexist manifestations)."

This seemingly innocent request sowed the seeds of much discord when the FQN sought to ban Miss Nude contests, erotic lingerie shows, royal family competitions, and politically incorrect street names in some of the clubs. At its November 1981 annual meeting the FQN adopted a protocol condemning such contests "where the roundest buns and the largest breasts see themselves rewarded with shiny trophies," on the grounds that naturism should include everyone without regard to physical development and should exclude "voyeurism, sexism, and the superiority/inferiority complexes which are conveyed by consumer society."[44]

Five clubs accepted these terms in 1983: Bel Air, Cyprès, Loisir Air Soleil, Oasis, and La Pommerie. Those who did not sign on— the "dinosaurs of naturism"—were mocked for their "paradisiacal vision" of "treeless trailer parks" where latter-day "Adams and Eves" could frolic in a "Garden of Eden." More and more the FQN pushed its version of naturism ever more strongly on the clubs, while moving towards the day when all club members would be required to join the Federation. This led the clubs to reconsider the advantages of affiliation—which seemed to consist of ever-increasing swarms of singles, whom they regarded simply as voyeurs (particularly the ones with cameras)—and one by one they withdrew from cooperation with the FQN.[45]

The mid-1980s marked the high point of FQN success.

Individual memberships topped 1,500; winter swims in Montreal, Quebec, and other cities attracted hundreds of devotees regularly; the magazine *Au Naturel* sold in public newsstands; FQN spokespersons appeared regularly in the media; and in 1985 the Federation moved into its brand new office in the Olympic Stadium. It was truly the "golden age" of the Federation. It also started a long, slow decline in FQN fortunes.

Membership in the FQN waxed and waned throughout the decade. One factor that was both cause and effect of declining membership, and of declining involvement in FQN activities, was the loss of all regional chapters outside Montreal. Even within Montreal the FQN lacked broad appeal, being—and wanting to be—limited to middle-aged, middle class professionals with a self-styled elitism that alienated club owners, members, and prospects alike. The esoteric interests of the leaders in astrology, yoga, and reflexology failed to appeal to rank and file members or to applicants.

> Naturists like to say about nudists that there is an equation: nudism = sex. But if you want to talk about equations, one could formulate one for naturists: naturism = belief that all known sciences are lies and that all pseudo-sciences are completely true.[46]

This esoteric elitism became the topic of a satire on the FQN published in *CROC*, Quebec's answer to *MAD* magazine. In its August 1989 issue *CROC* featured the "Quebec Bare Naked Federation" and its controversial former president, "Gerry Hardon." A parody of *Au Naturel*, here styled as "The New-dist" (with its special advisor Maharish-nude), told about the scouting origins of nudism with "Barebelly Powell" and presented a travel guide to "Nude York"; a review of recent films including "The Gods Must Have Fallen on Their Backsides," "The Accidental Nudist," and "Who Has Seen the Skin of Roger Rabbit?"; and a profile of prominent Quebec personalities like Jacques Parizeau wearing a strategic *fleur de lys* and nothing else.[47]

The deficit continued to climb despite generous donations

from members, but stringent economic measures helped eliminate the deficit—but not before the "precarious situation" of the FQN prompted some Federation members to set up a fall-back organization, the Fondation Naturiste du Québec, to "accumulate and administer a fund for the promotion of naturism."[48]

Fortunately the FQN survived the crisis and emerged leaner and meaner, continuing its publicity work—including regular seminars at the Olympic Stadium for previously neglected groups such as youths and anglophones (who had their own Montreal Association of Naturists in the late 1980s); participation in the 1992 Heritage Video, *Canada Naturally*; and a revamped *Au Naturel* in 1995 (followed in 2001 by its replacement, *Naturisme Québec*, published by the FQN founder)—and also improved relations with clubs by tacitly dropping its claims to tell them what to do and whom to admit. Although the founding president said in a retrospective interview on the fifteenth anniversary of the FQN that he would do the same thing over again—"I'm crazy enough for that!"—he added that "maybe I would have been a little more diplomatic." With both sides pulling back a little, they gained ground for compromise and cooperation.[49]

$\mathcal{N}udism\ \mathcal{T}oday$

In the past sixty years nudism in Canada has come full circle. What started as a natural, spontaneous recreational lifestyle among thousands of individuals in all parts of the country continues today as a way of life that appeals to the many people who seek natural recreation as the only truly satisfying respite from the storm and stress of life in the asphalt jungle.

In the sixties nudism took a quantum leap forward. The greater affluence of society led club members to demand better facilities and activities, and a new generation of parks and resorts emerged to cater to this demand. The sexual revolution produced greater public awareness of and tolerance for alternative ways of life, while encouraging more people to participate in those alternate lifestyles—particularly those involving nudity and nude recreation.

> Perhaps the increasing public acceptance of nudes (as distinct from nudism) has given us all a feeling of confidence (we still say that *Playboy* magazine has done more for the nudist movement than is generally admitted) but there is no doubt that the confidence is there.[1]

Likewise, the youth counterculture contributed to the social acceptance of nudism by its simple, nonchalant attitude towards being nude and natural. The decade of Woodstock (the real one) abounded in sit-ins, love-ins, be-ins, and occasional nude-ins—including the 1970 event that put Wreck Beach on the map. The new generation believed in everyone's right to live their own life without regard for the values of others who were not part of the lifestyle (a classic example being the skinny dipping nude-in at Mosport in 1970), and this changed the attitude of nudists towards nudism and the attitude of society towards both.[2]

The 1960s changed the content as well as the context of nudism through the emergence of naturism—or, more accurately, naturisms. On the one hand there are the libertarian individualists who "have no particular principles or philosophy, and exist mostly to promote hedonism and self-indulgence." On the other hand there is a more philosophical kind of naturism for "nudists who think" that accepts the physical freedom of nude recreation and the social ambience of non-sexist family nudism but situates people "a step back closer to nature" in the context of human respect for the global ecosystem. Or, in the words of the International Naturist Federation, naturism is "a way of living in harmony with nature, characterized by the practice of social nudity, with the intention of encouraging respect for oneself, respect for others, and care for the environment."[3]

The success of Canada's free beaches attests to the popularity of naturism. It also attests to the limited appeal of nudist clubs. Although there are dozens of well-established clubs in Canada, Wreck Beach alone outdraws all of them on any good summer weekend. Until fairly recently all Canadian clubs and organizations—from the original Canadian Sunbathing Association of 1947 to the later Eastern and Western Canadian Sunbathing Associations—stressed the safety, security, legality, and bureaucracy of small private clubs. Since the 1960s, however, more and more people prefer the natural spontaneity of free beach areas at home and abroad. The older clubs and organizations have reluctantly conceded this point.

> Last night we interviewed a middle-aged couple, prospective members. They had first encountered nudism last summer at Wreck Beach while on vacation in Vancouver, and were dismayed to learn that its freedom came about, not by the dedication of organ-

ized, respectable nudists but by the unorganized youngsters. They did not consider this to be to our credit.[4]

During the 1980s and 1990s nudism underwent yet another transition. Club membership remained static or even declined, while freelance naturism à la Wreck Beach increased in popularity, as did nude and clothing optional vacations in Europe and the Caribbean. The fate of the clubs reflected the aging of the owners and continuing turnover in membership. This has always been a feature of social nudism, as people try it out for a season or two and then lose interest, become disillusioned, or simply incorporate nudism into their everyday life and drop the social dimension of club life. But in the 1980s these traditional factors became compounded by the worsening economy, worsening weather patterns, and worsening news about ozone and melanoma.

On the other hand, the stresses and strains of life in the fast lane compels more and more people to escape the city for the peace and relaxation of the country. There is a growing market for rustic naturism (free beaches, swimming, sailing, camping, canoeing) without the sounds that abound in commercial vacation centers with their powerboats, ghetto blasters, and ubiquitous cell phones, and without the sanitized recreation of the larger nudist clubs where life seems to revolve around the bar more than the pool or the volleyball court.

One new type of camp eschewed traditional nudism in favor of clothing-optional recreation—today a fast-growing sector of the vacation market. During the 1970s a private forest reserve in the Haliburton Highlands offered clothing optional campsites on one of its thirteen secluded lakes surrounded by 90,000 wooded acres. In the 1980s a fishing lodge on Georgian Bay "shows the way to clothing optionality in the backwoods. The area is fine for fishing and canuding, hiking or boating in the buff, exploring the many rock formations and inlets." And in the 1990s a trailer park on Manitoulin Island reserved a section of its campground for nudists, while in eastern Ontario the Black River Country Inn offered "an intimate clothes-free bed and breakfast in a private, peaceful country setting."[5]

At the end of the 1980s several new landed clubs appeared in Ontario, organized by veteran nudists with extensive experience in established clubs, but targeted to a new generation. John Beddows, a newly retired schoolteacher in North Bay and former member of Norhaven, decided to re-create a "wilderness for naturists" on a private lake midway between North Bay and Sturgeon Falls. Jewel Lake Wilderness offers one square mile of untouched pine forest surrounding the 100 acre Cockburn Lake—an ideal setting for camping, fishing, canoeing, and windsurfing, along with bird, moose, and deer watching: "an opportunity for Toronto and other urban naturists to experience a true northern adventure!"[6] At the same time three veterans of Lakesun, residents of Ottawa, decided to start their own club and acquired 500 acres of land surrounding Jameson Lake near Calabogie, about one hour west of Ottawa. Like Jewel Lake, Sunward offers rustic camping centering around the lake, with swimming, fishing, canoeing, and windsurfing. "Of course, we have the obligatory family of loons and an abundance of other flora and fauna. You and your children are welcome to explore the lake and surrounding forest, pick the flowers, and catch frogs if you like."[7]

Another round of nudist development started in the 1990s with the emergence of three non-landed travel clubs, which offer an informal framework in which people can enjoy a broad range of nudist activities on a year-round basis without requiring full-time membership in one specific landed club.[8]

The Ontario Roaming Bares (ORB), originally based in Toronto, organizes group activities, including visits to Glen Echo, Ponderosa, and Four Seasons; outings to beaches, isolated lakes, and hiking trails; and trips to regional Naturist Society gatherings in the U.S. Starting in 1995 ORB sponsored successful indoor swims at a Toronto municipal pool. Unlike other groups in other cities, ORB arranged to offer these monthly swim nights year-round because "city naturists, like all naturists, enjoy skinny dipping in the summer and need a pool that is close to home and public transit."[9]

The Ottawa Naturists/Naturistes de l'Outaouais (ON/NO) are the first Canadian nudist club formed via e-mail. Given easy access to Meech Lake and several landed clubs, they decided that their priority should be indoor winter activity, specifically swimming. ON/NO arranged to rent a municipal pool from the city of Ottawa. Besides splashing around in the pool, ON/NO held bimonthly social meetings to present information, slides, and videos on naturist vacation opportunities in Ontario, Quebec, the United States, and "warm locations." During the summer months the club organizes group trips to East Haven, Lakesun, Sunward, and the Grand Barn, while individuals travel to American locations summer and winter.[10]

The third travel club is the Northern Sunbirds Association, which formed in Thunder Bay in 1993. The Lakehead area had been home to an earlier club, but the impetus for the Sunbirds was the relocation to Thunder Bay of Terry Hill, a former FCN president whose family had belonged to Glen Echo. A local ad in the paper brought several people to a public seminar, and some of them joined the group's outings to "a remote lake with a beautiful beach." Like the Ottawa Naturists, the Northern Sunbirds alternate business and social meetings, including winter saunas. Summer activities include visits to Crocus Grove in Winnipeg, joint trips with a U.S. naturist group in Duluth, and—starting in 1995—use of their own landed base, Tylara Hills, west of Thunder Bay.[11]

Several recent landed clubs offer their own unique appeal to travellers. On the expressway from Ottawa to Montreal the Grand Barn offers a clothing-optional haven for naturists, naturalists, musicians, artists, and anyone else who appreciates a "new age" ambience. At the opposite end of Ontario, Hidden Lakes Resort's "clothing optional environment allows you to just be yourself" (unless you are a single male, in which case admission "is at the discretion of the management"). Appropriately enough, this newest club lies near Minaki Lodge, where Ontario nudism began.[12]

In eastern Canada the Sunny Vale Nature Park opened in June 1991. A year earlier, several nudists in Nova Scotia, patrons of free beaches, formed the Maritimes Organized Naturist Association (MONA), which reorganized in 1991 as the Federation of Atlantic Naturists (FAN). One couple, Scott and Pauline, decided that the time was ripe for a landed club and created Sunny Vale on 100 acres of bushland. In 1993, in an effort to boost attendance above 100 visits per season, Sunny Vale organized an Atlantic Naturist Gathering, but with limited success. Prospective members were deterred by the exclusive proprietary management of the club, the limited facilities, and its excessive secrecy, reflected in frequent changes of address and phone number and the club's pledge (or threat) to screen all applicants through the "Canadian Police Information Center." The club subsequently folded.[13]

The Bluenose Naturist Club, formed by beachgoers and former Sunny Vale members in 1991, is much more active. Originally started to defend Crystal Crescent Beach against threats from police and real-estate developers, Bluenose evolved into a typical non-landed club by organizing indoor winter swims in Halifax, by hosting group parties, and by maintaining a continued presence on "their" beach, including semi-annual beach sweeps to clean up refuse.[14]

In the BC Interior, where individuals have always been able to get "all the privacy they want for going in the nude by taking a short walk from the village," a few clubs appeared over the years to bring nudists together—especially when the "villages" turned into an "up and coming summer resort" or a city. In 1960 an enthusiastic couple in Kamloops started the Kam Tans. Boasting of "the nicest weather in Canada," the Kam Tans relied on local newspaper advertising to attract applicants. But the response was insufficient to keep the club going. Two later clubs in the Okanagan were more successful, and both depended on outsiders with club experience who transferred to the valley on business. In the mid-1960s a Calgary businessman moved to Penticton and started the Sunny Mainliners. Although this was a travel club which arranged group outings and winter parties, one member made his land available for sunning and swimming. But when the founder transferred back to Calgary, the club folded.[15]

In 1989 Merv Krull, founder of the Edmonton Nudist Society, relocated to Salmon Arm, BC, and promptly founded the Okanagan-Shuswap Nudist Society to serve nudists in the BC interior by providing "places for families and couples to spend relaxing quality time away from the stresses and demands of everyday living." The club affiliated with the WCSA, the Federation of Canadian Naturists, and the Naturist Society. Members enjoy indoor winter swims and outdoor summer trips to nearby nude beaches. They also pioneered popular houseboat cruises on Shuswap Lake. In 1993 the Salmon Arm group spawned its own offshoot, the Kelowna Nudist Club, which hosts monthly swim nights. And in 1994 the founders bought land near Vernon for a permanent landed campground to serve the Okanagan Valley.[16]

The Federation of Canadian Naturists (FCN)—an organization based like the Quebec Federation of Naturism on individual rather than club memberships—was born in 1985 but was conceived several years earlier in the minds of a "self-appointed committee" of three members of the Glen Echo club: Doug and Helen Beckett, who had experience with the older ECSA/CNC and with the WCSA during a work stint out west, and Petra Scheller, of the younger generation but a lifelong and enthusiastic naturist. Occasional discussion and reminiscences about the "good old days" led them to think about a new organization to unite all Canadian nudists and promote naturism to the general public.[17]

These early FCN activists knew that they were not working in a vacuum. They were aware of the WCSA and of the FQN. Since they shared a sympathy for naturism and a desire for a Canadian organization, they first contacted the FQN in Montreal. Michel Vais, founder and vice-president, recounted his experience in Quebec and offered advice which they gratefully accepted. One result of this FQN input was that the FCN became a member-based rather than a club-based organization (something that would later complicate its discussions with the WCSA). Besides, the historical record of both the ECSA and WCSA demonstrated the limitations inherent in club-based organizations, whereas the FQN already had more members after one decade than the WCSA had after four decades.[18]

In 1985 things began to gel. The volunteers reconstituted themselves and elected a founding committee, which continued contacts with other clubs and organizations and started to work on a constitution. In 1986 Petra Scheller, already acting as public relations director, visited western Canada and contacted the Wreck Beach Preservation Society. Later that year she attended the WCSA convention in Calgary after Tom Dunn of the WCSA had visited Glen Echo to discuss relations between the two organizations. Dunn remained sympathetic to the FCN and would later serve on the its board.[19]

The FCN is set up as a federation of individual members (clubs may join as corporate individuals). Originally it was a national organization that included local members from different regions of Canada on the board of directors, but conflicts of jurisdiction with the erstwhile mentor FQN, differences of opinion with the WCSA, and difficulties in recruiting regional members and directors led to a restructuring in 1990 which made the FCN into a congeries of four regional mini-FCNs united under one national umbrella. But in practice this framework simply superimposed the possibility of regional organizations on the original federal outline. The FCN remains a nationwide organization with five members of the board serving as president, vice president, secretary, treasurer, and public relations officer, and with two members representing each of the four regions of Canada: British Columbia, the Yukon, and the Northwest Territories; the prairie provinces of Alberta, Saskatchewan, and Manitoba; the central provinces of Ontario and Quebec (with due regard for the primary responsibility of the FQN for the francophone population of Quebec); and the Atlantic provinces. At the 1995 annual meeting FCN members formally established a separate board of directors for the Central Region to reflect the rapid growth of new clubs in Ontario.[21]

In defining its relationship with the other regions of Canada the FCN immediately encountered two other well-established regional organizations, which were not about to surrender their autonomy, particularly since both the WCSA and the FQN long preceded the FCN, and the WCSA still bitterly remembered the role of eastern Canadians in destroying the previous national organization—the Canadian Sunbathing Association: "we are still growing upward and onward, which is more than the E.C.S.A. ever did. . . . It is indeed unfortunate that the bitterness of what did take place some years ago, has left its mark for so many years." So the FCN had its work cut out when it set its regional framework in regions which already had active nudist organizations.[22]

The principal issue between the FCN and the FQN concerned Canada's representation in the International Naturist Federation (INF), a European-based, worldwide association of national nudist organizations that is affiliated with UNESCO. The FQN held Canada's seat in the INF formerly occupied by the CNC until its demise in 1978; the FCN, perhaps prematurely, thought that it should hold that seat as the only national Canadian organization (the WCSA was content to ride on the INF coattails of the ASA); and the INF forced a confrontation, because its new rules required that only one organization could represent any one country. To resolve their differences the two federations created a permanent liaison committee, the Union FQN-FCN/FQN-FCN Union, in 1988. The union is a creation of the executive boards of the two federations for the purpose of joint liaison and representation to the INF. It cannot say or do anything without unanimous consent and the approval of both executive boards. Expenses on joint projects are shared equally, and the two federations alternately designate their official delegates to the INF congresses.[23]

Ironically, the accord between the FCN and the FQN helped doom the FCN's approach to the other established Canadian organization, the WCSA, because westerners resented the fact that, like Ottawa, the FCN was obligated to "rubber stamp" everything that Quebec wanted, and because they naively assumed that "C comes before Q." However, the FCN had an important selling point: it was a Canadian organization—despite its "misguided" insistence on naturism instead of nudism—and would be more likely than the fraternal ASA to be informed on and involved with Canadian affairs, and more likely to collect dues in Canadian dollars. For its part the "fraternal" ASA indicated that it "would not stand in the way if the WCSA decides to switch to the FCN."[24]

The FCN's equally limited success with the clubs prompted a new strategy. It began approaching Ontario nudist clubs in 1987. But for awhile the suitor seemed less interested than the courted. When these early attempts at outreach brought limited results at the expense of even more limited resources, the FCN reappraised its policy and created a form of "club membership," in which a club could become a member of the FCN as a corporate individual without prejudice to the affiliation of the club's own members.[25]

Once the FCN realized the limits of top-down growth through affiliation with clubs and other organizations, it decided to focus on "educating and informing the public on the naturist lifestyle and as a by-product get more members." Publicity was the way to go. Feature articles, interviews, and reports on clubs, beaches, and vacation destinations appeared in major Ontario newspapers, while Petra Scheller and other representatives appeared on local and national radio talkshows. When the FCN sponsored a screening of the ASA promotional video "Welcome to Our World" on cable TV in Toronto one Etobicoke viewer cried foul, but the OPP reported that "there was nothing objectionable and that it was a well-presented topic."[26]

Perhaps the most successful—because understated and unsolicited—PR event was a nation-wide television commercial for the Sears Club in early 1991. The ad depicted several ordinary social groups and clubs going about their everyday business in one scene and endorsing the Sears Club in another. Among these normal, everyday groups was the "Nature's Way Nudist Club" of Prince Edward Island, who were depicted nude (albeit behind a strategic banner). The whole scene was handled tastefully and presented naturism as an ordinary, everyday way of life. It was not, unfortunately, regarded as natural and ordinary in Charlottetown, where a spokesman for Anne of Green Gables avowed that "the Island is noted for its wholesomeness." The province in fact had no such club (although there is a nude beach at Blooming Point), and that is why Sears placed its fictional club there.[27] More recently a Reactine commercial portrayed relief from allergies by showing a young man disrobing in a forest glen and romping around the flowers in his newfound freedom to the tune of Air Supply's "All I Need Is the Air That I Breathe," and to the bemusement of some little old ladies inspecting the flora and fauna with magnifying glasses.

Public seminars represent a form of publicity intermediate between the scatter-shot press releases in the general media and the more specific displays at nudist conventions and clubs. Media publicity informs people about the existence of nudist clubs and organizations ready to provide further information. But for those individuals who have already thought about nude recreation and think that it might be for them, small-group public seminars provide a more practical introduction to social nudism, more specific answers to first-time questions and concerns, and more precise information about the types of clubs and beaches in the area, and about the steps necessary to visit or to join them.[28]

To further promote social nudism to the public, the FCN accepted a suggestion from the FQN in 1987 to produce a bilingual *Canadian Guide to Nudist Clubs and Beaches*, which proved popular enough to justify subsequent editions. The two federations also cooperated with David Ball and Heritage Videos to produce the two-part *Canada Naturally* video in 1992. Although this year had one of the wettest summers on record, the team found enough sunny days to produce film portraits of eleven clubs in Ontario and Quebec. Many of the scenes were captured in the book *Canada Naturally* by Richard West.[29]

In 1996 the FCN sponsored the Young Canadian Naturists (YCN) group to reach young singles and retain their interest in nudism. The YCN advertised in student newspapers, while spokespeople appeared on university and college radio stations. They also prepared a pamphlet for teens touting the "Top 15 Way Cool Reasons to Spend a Day or a Weekend at a Nudist Campground/Beach." But the organizers found—as have their counterparts in the Junior Division of the American Association for Nude Recreation—that most of the young singles have left the clubs by age 18 and aren't available for organizing. Europeans have more success with generational outreach, but they start with younger age groups and provide a greater variety of all-youth activities.[30]

Rather than giving up hope, the YCN redirected its focus from teens to twens, particularly university students and young professionals. The group drew on the success of the newly formed Ontario Roaming Bares, whose monthly swim nights at municipal pools in Toronto attracted large numbers of young singles and couples. YCN spun off the University of Toronto Naturists, who took advantage of the Hart House Farm in the Caledon Hills. UTN in turn inspired the Naturists of Waterloo. All of these groups remain small, but clearly fill a niche in contemporary nudism.[31]

In 1999 the FCN commissioned a public opinion survey to determine public attitudes towards nudism. The results were encouraging: 20 per cent of respondents said that they have skinny-dipped or visited a nude beach, or would do so given the opportunity; 40 per cent said they have experienced or would consider domestic nudity around the house; and 60 per cent have slept nude or would consider doing so. The results suggested policy for the future: more media publicity, more seminars, more assistance for new clubs and groups, more support for nude beaches and nude recreation, more cooperation among all Canadian organizations, and in general more work "to further the understanding and acceptance of naturism so that anyone, anywhere in Canada, will be able to enjoy nude recreation both in clubs and on public beaches without fear of arrest or harassment."[32]

From a nucleus of three volunteers in 1985, the FCN has grown into a nation-wide organization with some two thousand members. Over the years the FCN has created an organization that spans the whole of Canada, embracing all ten provinces, and has established close ties with two regional organizations, the FQN and the WCANR, as well as with the Wreck Beach Preservation Society. The federation's quarterly magazine, *Going Natural*, has received special recognition from the International Naturist Federation, and the FCN maintains an active public relations presence in the media (including Internet and World Wide Web access) and with government tourism offices. In 2000 it acquired a permanent office and library at the Glen Echo club near Toronto.[33]

In the best of all possible worlds people should be free to enjoy a nude and natural way of life in any appropriate context. Downtown Vancouver or Toronto or Montreal may not be appropriate (unlike downtown Munich), but in a country the size of Canada, with millions of square miles of woodland, hundreds of thousands of lakes, and hundreds of miles of ocean beaches and Great Lakes shores, there is certainly room for nude and natural recreation. Until that happens on a greater scale than at present, Canadians will continue to travel abroad in search of the freedom that should be theirs at home. Cuba, Guadeloupe, Jamaica, and St Martin, and are just a few of the Caribbean islands that lure Canadian sun bunnies to the "magic and adventure" of clothing optional beaches.

> There I was on the island of Curaçao feeling the breeze on my chest. It was the first time ever I had bared my breasts.
>
> I noticed that nobody cared if I uncovered my breasts, let alone if they were big or small, pointy or sagging. Knowing this made me feel at ease.
>
> I noticed that both men and women were really cool about this baring of breasts. Women did not show off or flaunt their torsos. And men did not stare. Both

sexes, all of different ages, were relaxed and carefree. Wow!

I knew that this was truly a vacation, and that all of its magic and adventure would soon be gone.[34]

What organized nudism and nudist organizations have tried to do throughout their history is to bring this sense of magic and adventure home—to encourage and enable Canadians to enjoy a nude and natural lifestyle in one of the greatest natural countries anywhere. But despite more than sixty years of effort naturism in Canada (and in the United States) lags well behind the participation rate in Europe. The Netherlands alone, with half as many people as Canada on territory a fraction the size of Canada, has far more nudists than either Canada or the United States. North Americans have long lamented this discrepancy, which is due in part to differences in history—the broad social consensus in postwar Europe on achieving a better quality of life for all, in contrast to the North American obsession with achieving a better material standard of living for those who can afford it—and partly structural, since the centralized European states can implement social policies on a national scale without the incumbrance of federal politics. The one thing that European, American, and Canadian proponents of nudism have going for them is the unrelenting stress and congestion of life in an urbanized, industrialized, commercialized, materialized society. As long as that "lifestyle" is with us, there will be people who will want a breath of fresh air—all over.

INDEX
To Beaches, Clubs, Organizations, and Publications